# Pharmacogenomics and Pharmacogenetics in Drug Therapy

*Edited by Madhu Khullar, Anupam Mittal and Amol Patil*

Published in London, United Kingdom

Pharmacogenomics and Pharmacogenetics in Drug Therapy
http://dx.doi.org/10.5772/intechopen.107765
Edited by Madhu Khullar, Anupam Mittal and Amol Patil

Contributors
Abdul Hafeez, Adalberto Rezende Santos, Afreen Usmani, Anupam Mittal, Ashok Pavithra, Cecilia Alvim Dutra, Charul Jain, Georges Nemer, Harrison Magdinier Gomes, Madhu Khullar, Mohammad Khalid, Mohd Aftab Siddiqui, Mohd Mujahid, Márcia Quinhones P. Lopes, Nagham Nafiz Hendi, Philip Noel Suffys, Raquel Lima De Figueiredo Lima de F. Teixeira, Reddy Amala, Sairam Venkatraman, Srinivasan S. Tharun, Victória Moraes-Silva



First published in London, United Kingdom, 2024 by IntechOpen
IntechOpen is the global imprint of INTECHOPEN LIMITED, registered in England and Wales, registration number: 11086078, 167-169 Great Portland Street, London, W1W 5PF, United Kingdom

British Library Cataloguing-in-Publication Data
A catalogue record for this book is available from the British Library

Additional hard and PDF copies can be obtained from orders@intechopen.com

Pharmacogenomics and Pharmacogenetics in Drug Therapy
Edited by Madhu Khullar, Anupam Mittal and Amol Patil
p. cm.

This title is part of the Pharmaceutical Science Book Series, Volume 3
Topic: Pharmacology
Series Editor: Rosario Pignatello
Topic Editor: Cristina Manuela Drăgoi
Associate Topic Editor: Alina Crenguţa Nicolae

Print ISBN 978-1-83768-526-4
Online ISBN 978-1-83768-527-1
eBook (PDF) ISBN 978-1-83768-528-8
ISSN 3033-3318

For EU product safety concerns:
IN TECH d.o.o., Prolaz Marije Krucifikse Kozulić 3, 51000 Rijeka, Croatia,
info@intechopen.com or visit our website at intechopen.com.

IntechOpen Book Series

# Pharmaceutical Science

Volume 3

## Aims and Scope of the Series

Pharmaceutical science focuses on the design, synthesis, formulation, targeting, distribution, safety, and efficacy of active compounds as potential therapeutics. It is a large interdisciplinary discipline that aims to integrate the basic principles of physical and organic chemistry, biochemistry, biology, and engineering to discover, develop, and characterize active compounds and to optimize the formulation and delivery of drugs in the body for offering new and improved safe and efficacious therapies against human diseases. The research areas covered by the pharmaceutical sciences range from medicinal chemistry and pharmaceutical technology to pharmacology and toxicology, which represent the preliminary phases of drug development. Medicinal chemistry involves the design and synthesis of pharmaceuticals as well as the isolation of active agents from natural sources. Computer-aided strategies are increasingly involved in this drug discovery process. Pharmaceutics is a multidisciplinary science that examines the relationships between drug formulation, delivery, distribution, and clinical outcomes. Modern clinical approaches are increasingly relying on controlled release strategies and drug delivery and targeting systems, including nanotechnological platforms (nanomedicine). Pharmacology is the science of drug action in biological systems. Pharmacologists also make drugs as tools to explore aspects of cell and tissue functions. Toxicology is the study of the adverse effects of active agents on living organisms and the ecosystem, including the prevention and amelioration of such adverse effects. This book series includes volumes on Drug Discovery, Delivery, and Pharmacology. Their overall aim is to present the latest research in the whole path of drug discovery and development from different points of view of this multidisciplinary and dynamic field.

# Meet the Series Editor

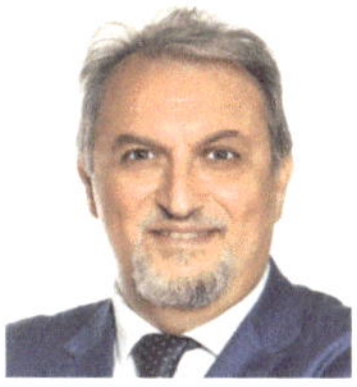

Prof. Rosario Pignatello is a Full Professor of Pharmaceutical Technology and Legislation at the University of Catania, Italy. He is the Director of the Department of Drug and Health Sciences. He has nearly 30 years of experience in the research and development of innovative formulations for the controlled release and targeting of bioactive molecules, through chemical approaches as well as nanotechnological carriers, aimed at treating different disorders. Prof. Pignatello has coauthored about 180 papers and edited a series of textbooks on biomaterials and their application in medicine. The main areas of his research are polymeric and lipid-based micro- and nanoparticles as modified drug delivery systems; vesicular nanocarriers (liposomes, micelles); lipophilic prodrugs and conjugates; synthesis and evaluation of new polymeric biomaterials for drug delivery and tissue regeneration. In particular, Prof. Pignatello works actively in the field of ocular drug delivery, leading the Research Centre for Ocular Nanotechnology, within the NANOMED Centre (Centre for Nanomedicine and Pharmaceutical Nanotechnology) at the University of Catania.

# Meet the Volume Editor

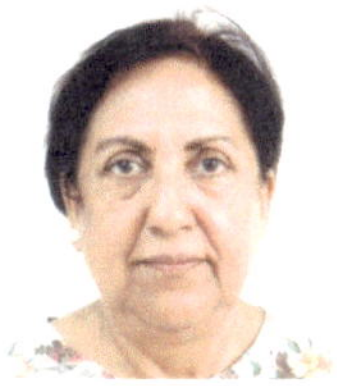

Dr. Madhu Khullar, Ph.D., is an ex-professor of the Department of Experimental Medicine and Biotechnology, Post Graduate Institute of Medical Education and Research, Chandigarh, India. She was an emeritus scientist of the Indian Council of Medical Education and Research, India. She is a fellow in hypertension research from Henry Ford Hospital, Detroit, USA, and was the recipient of the Fogarty Fellowship, NIH, USA and the Department of Biotechnology overseas fellowship in genetics research. She is a fellow of the National Academy of Medical Sciences, India; a fellow of the International Academy of Cardiovascular Research, and a fellow of the International Society of Nutrition. She has a keen research interest in molecular mechanisms, genetics, and functional genomics of cardiovascular diseases, including cardiomyopathies, hypertension, and diabetic nephropathy. She has published nearly 200 research papers in peer-reviewed journals, edited several books and contributed chapters in various books.

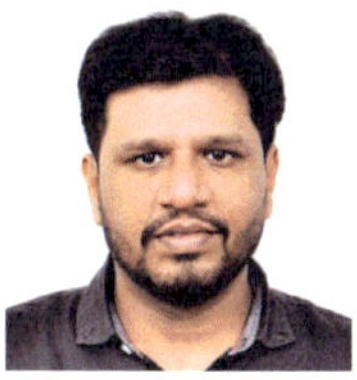

Dr. Anupam Mittal, Ph.D., has been an assistant professor in the Department of Translational and Regenerative Medicine since 2019. He is a member of various prestigious scientific bodies. He has a keen research interest in the genetics and functional genomics of cardiovascular diseases, including cardiomyopathies, congenital heart diseases, and cardio-renal syndrome. He also has an interest in pluripotent stem cells as a drug discovery and repurposing model. He has a good track record in the field of cardiovascular biology. He has contributed to various publications and book chapters in the field.

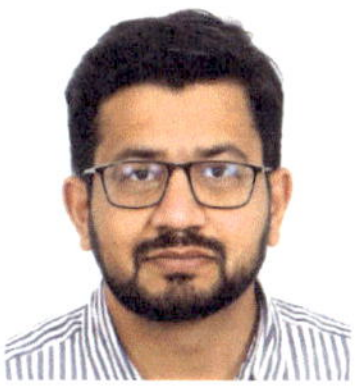

Dr. Amol Patil is currently working as an additional professor and is in charge of drug information center services in the Department of Pharmacology, PGIMER, Chandigarh. He obtained his primary medical education, namely an MBBS, from Seth G S Medical College and KEM Hospital, Mumbai. Dr. Patil pursued his career in clinical pharmacology as an MD and DM, as his prime interest lies in pharmacogenetics and personalized medicine. He has developed several patient services for tailoring the medication doses. He has two patents, over 80 research papers in national and international journals, and book chapters to his credit.

# Contents

# Preface

There is a wide variation in the drug response of different individuals. Until recently, drug therapeutics was based on average pharmacokinetic data collected by response to a particular drug in a group of people. Such approaches often resulted in adverse drug reactions or inept drug responses in individuals of different ethnic groups. Pharmacogenomics involves the study of variations in the genome (DNA polymorphisms) and changes in RNA characteristics as related to drug response, and pharmacogenetics addresses the role of genetic variations in drug response. Both pharmacogenetics and pharmacogenomics are very effective tools in the field of precision medicine. Precision medicine personalizes medical treatment based on the patient's genetic makeup and the way their body processes a particular drug at biological and molecular levels. It helps in minimizing adverse drug reactions and optimizing drug responsiveness at a personalized level.

This book provides recent literature on the role of genetic variants in drug response in some drug therapies. It includes an introductory chapter giving an overview of the role of pharmacogenomics and pharmacogenetics of various drug therapies in different diseases such as cardiovascular disease, psychiatric disorders, and cancers. The book also includes chapters on the pharmacogenetics of aspirin, type 2 diabetes, the human Nat2 gene, and cardiovascular diseases.

**Madhu Khullar**
Ex Professor,
Department of Experimental Medicine and Biotechnology,
Post Graduate Institute of Medical Education and Research,
Chandigarh, India

**Anupam Mittal**
Assistant Professor,
Department of Translational and Regenerative Medicine,
Post Graduate Institute of Medical Education and Research,
Chandigarh, India

**Amol Patil**
Department of Pharmacology,
Post Graduate Institute of Medical Education and Research,
Chandigarh, India

Chapter 1

# Introductory Chapter: Pharmacogenomics and Pharmacogenetics in Drug Therapy

*Anupam Mittal and Madhu Khullar*

## 1. Introduction

There is a wide variation in drug response of different individuals of different ethnic groups. Till recently, drug therapeutics was based on average pharmacokinetic data collected by response to a particular drug in a group of people. Such approach, many a times resulted, in adverse drug reactions, or inept drug response in individuals of different ethnic groups. In fact, adverse drug reactions (ADRs) have been reported to be a major cause of hospitalization and mortality worldwide. Also, the treatment for several diseases such as hypertension, depression etc. is still empirical as it is based on hit and trial, resulting in delays in effective treatment and high cost. The variability in drug response has been attributed to race, ethnicity, poor compliance, lack of target specificity of drug and drug-drug interactions.

Pharmacogenomics refers to the application of genomics information of an individual in determining how genome of an individual may respond to treatment with a particular drug. On the other hand, the term 'Pharmacogenetics' refers to the role that genes of an individual play in determining drug response of that individual. According to world-wide pharmacological consortium, 'Pharmacogenomics' involves the study of variations in genome (DNA polymorphisms) and changes in RNA characteristics as related to drug response, and 'Pharmacogenetics' addresses the role of genetic variations in relation to drug response [1]. Both pharmacogenetics and pharmacogenomics are very effective tools in the field of precision medicine. Precision medicine personalizes the medical treatment based on patient's genetic makeup and the way, body processes a particular drug at biological and molecular levels. It helps in minimizing adverse drug reactions and optimizing drug responsiveness at personalized level. It is a rapidly expanding area of research with wide translational applications in drug therapies for various diseases such as cardiovascular diseases, renal diseases, cancer, hypertension, and mental health.

With the rapid progress in Next generation sequencing techniques like microarray, transcriptomics and whole exome sequencing, choice of drug therapy is now increasingly made based on genetic profiling, lifestyle, and environmental factors. The major limitation of current usage of pharmacogenomics is that it is being used in very few health conditions due to lack of availability of data for many diseases in different populations.

Pharmacokinetics and Pharmacodynamics of the drug are the two important components of drug response. Pharmacokinetics involve studying the role of factors such as drug absorption, metabolism, excretion etc. in determining the concentration of drug or its active metabolites. Pharmacodynamics of a drug addresses the interaction of the drug or its active metabolite with its target molecule(s) or its downstream effector molecules. Studies have shown that both pharmacogenomics and pharmacogenetics modulate pharmacodynamics and pharmacokinetics parameters of the associated drugs.

## 2. Role of genetic variations in drug response

Drug concentration is an important factor which contributes to variable drug response. It has been observed that genetic variations such as single nucleotide polymorphisms (SNPs) and copy number variations (CNVs) in genes of drug metabolizing and transport enzymes can significantly modulate drug concentrations. For example, polymorphism in *CYP2C19* gene has been shown to modulate clopidrogel response, while polymorphism in CYP2C9 gene alters warfarin response by altering its pharmacokinetic parameters. On the other hand, polymorphism in *CYP4F2* gene has been shown to modulate pharmacodynamics of warfarin [2]. The *CYP2C19* metabolizes clopidrogel to its bioactive compound and this depends on its genetic variants. Homozygous variants for *CYP2C19*2* code for loss-of-function proteins which completely lack *CYP2C19* activity and thus are not good responders to warfarin. Heterozygous carriers, on other hand show response on increasing the dose as they possess some enzyme activity. Thus, response based on gene variants shows variability depending on the gene locus as well as genetic variant(s) at a particular locus.

Many effects of gene variants in drug metabolizing enzymes have been associated with gain or loss of function of the gene activity, with predominance linked to gain of function effect. This has been well described for increased copy numbers of CYP2D6, a morphine metabolizing enzyme, resulting in enhanced effect of morphine during codeine therapy [2].

Genetic variants of certain drug metabolizing enzymes may also increase susceptibility to drug toxicity by modulating its plasma concentrations. This is apparent in case of some drugs which show a very small margin between effective and toxic concentrations. Thus, a genetic variant may result in increased or decreased concentration of the active drug metabolite. For example, some of thiopurine S-methyltransferase (TPMT) gene variants have been reported to enhance toxicity of immunosuppressant drug, azathioprine. Toxicity of several anticancer drugs has also been shown to be influenced by polymorphisms in TPMT and other drug metabolizing enzymes [2]. Further, toxic effects of the gene variants are also dependent on how a specific drug is metabolized. It has been observed that those drugs which are metabolized by a single enzyme show less modulation by gene variants [2] and the drugs metabolized by multiple enzymes/pathways are not influenced by gene polymorphisms unless the polymorphism affect more than one enzyme of the drug metabolizing pathway [2]. Further genetic variations leading to loss or gain of function of genes coding for enzymes involved in drug transport into or out of a cell can also alter drug efficacy/response and sometimes its toxicity. This is seen in case of SNP SLCO1B1*5 of SLCO1B1 gene which results in loss of function leading to increased Simvastatin plasma levels and myopathy [2].

The ancestry has a big role in determining the response to a drug due to prevalence of certain genotypes in a specific community/race. Some genotypes affecting loss or gain of function of a gene involved in drug metabolism, or drug receptor interaction may be solely present in a particular population, thereby affecting drug response/toxicity or efficacy. For example, HLA-B*15:02 genotype is more prevalent in Southeast Asia and has been found to be associated with carbamazepine-related drug toxicity, however, this allele is rare in European population, leading to less adverse carbamazepine-related drug reactions [2].

## 3. Clinical applications of pharmacogenomics and pharmacogenetics

Due to availability of vast data supporting role of pharmacogenomics and pharmacogenetics in modulating response to drugs, several pre-clinical and clinical trials have been carried out in this direction. In February 2020, FDA published a 'Table of Pharmacogenetic Associations which provides clinically useful information on drug-gene interactions and their clinical outcomes [3]. This table provides detailed scientific evidence for genotype-phenotype associations of several clinical drugs. There is also detailed information on pharmacogenomics of drugs in clinical use compiled by Clinical Pharmacogenetics Implementation Consortium (CPIC) guidelines. These guidelines have also been annotated in Pharmacogenomics Knowledgebase [4].

The major applications of pharmacogenomics/genetics in the field of cardiovascular diseases, oncology, psychiatry, diabetes, antiretroviral and immunological therapies have been discussed in the subsequent chapters of this book.

### 3.1 Cardiovascular diseases

Antiplatelet drug, Clopidogrel is widely used in patients undergoing percutaneous coronary intervention (PCI). This drug is metabolized to its active compound in a two-step enzymatic reaction catalyzed by CYP2C19. Three gene variants of this enzyme, CYP2C19 *1/*2/*3 are associated with normal (*1) or loss of function (*2/*3) activity. This results in either normal metabolism (NM) or poor metabolism (PM) of the drug, resulting in varied drug availability in different genotypes. This results in increasing the risk of adverse events in *2 and *3 genotype carriers at normal doses. Tripling the drug dose in *2 and *3 genotype carriers has been found to be effective. Hence, it is now mandatory in several countries to genotype patients before prescribing this drug [5]. In fact, it is one of the most common pharmacogenetic applications in a clinical condition. Another drug, Warfarin, a vitamin K antagonist is used for treating thromboembolic disorders. This drug shows varied genotype-phenotype response, which is dependent on gene variants of *CYP2C9* and *VKORC1*. Another example is statins, which are commonly prescribed drugs in dyslipidaemia. In some patients, they can cause adverse drug reactions like myopathy, as in case of Simvastatin. The gene variants of *SLCO1B1* have been reported to be associated with this adverse reaction [6].

In addition to above drugs, there is emerging evidence of pharmacogenetic based response to β-blockers. β-blockers are commonly used drugs in hypertension and in heart diseases. They function by blocking β1-adrenergic receptor coded by the *ADRB1* gene. Two gene variants in ADRB1, Ser49Gly and Arg389Gly have been shown to be associated with increased adrenergic activity and increased mortality in patients treated with Verapamil [7]. β-blocker treatment in patients carrying these alleles has been found to reduce mortality and is recommended over calcium channel blockers. Several other ADRB1 gene variants have also been found to modulate response to β-blockers [7]. Polymorphisms in *GRK4* (G protein coupled receptor gene), have also been shown to modulate β blocker activity and associated cardiovascular outcomes. Polymorphisms in several other genes involved in mechanism/metabolism of β-blockers such as CYP2D6 are plausible candidate genes being explored for their effect on B blocker response [8]. Similarly, activity of ACE inhibitors, Angiotensin Type II receptor blockers (ARBs), diuretics etc. has been shown to be modulated by polymorphisms in genes associated with pharmacokinetics, pharmacodynamics, and metabolism of the target molecules.

### 3.2 Mental health disorders

Mental diseases such as depression, schizophrenia, anxiety are major health disorders associated with general morbidity, mortality, and disability worldwide. Research in the past decade has documented that treatment with antidepressant drugs is often not effective and may elicit varied response. This has been partly attributed to genetic factors, especially in the target genes of anti-psychotic drugs, namely *SLC6A4, HTR2A, HTR2C, DRD2, ABCB1, CYP2C19, CYP2D6,* and *COMT* genes which code for serotonin reuptake, transporters, dopamine D2 receptor, P-glycoprotein that control uptake of drugs into the brain and drug-metabolizing enzymes respectively. As reviewed recently, genetic polymorphisms in drug metabolizing genes *CYP2C19* and *CYP2D6* have maximal clinical application and patients are stratified into normal, intermediate, and poor metabolisers based on the carrier status of functional gene variants, which in turn determine the activity of the metabolizing enzymes. It has been observed that genotype affects the success of antidepressant or antipsychotic therapy in patients. It has been suggested that genotyping based dosing of patients receiving these drugs may result in better treatment response [9]. A recent systematic review has shown that blood levels of several drugs such as aripiprazole, haloperidol, risperidone, escitalopram, and sertraline were significantly associated genetic variants of *CYP2C19* and *CYP2D6* and could be a useful tool for precision drug dosing in patients [10]. However, it was concluded that more studies are needed for this to be implemented as a clinical tool. Thus, pharmacogenetics of psychiatric drugs has the potential to develop as a useful and cost-effective tool for precision medicine and compliance with minimal adverse effects.

### 3.3 Oncotherapy

Cancer is one of the major health concerns, prevalent in all the parts of the world. The major issue with the cancer treatment is due to prevalence of non-responders and relapse cases. As many as 75% of the cancer patients are non-responsive towards the conventional therapy [11]. For example, 5-fluorouracil is one of the most widely preferred therapy for colorectal and gastric cancer [12]. In the human liver cells, dihydropyrimidine dehydrogenase (DPD) is the main enzyme responsible for the metabolism of 5-fluorouracil [13]. DPD expression is the major gene which decides the response and the tolerability to 5-FU-based chemotherapy [12]. Previous studies have shown that four DPYD variants are very important, taking into consideration their impact on enzyme function and toxicity risk: rs3918290, rs55886062, rs67376798, and rs75017182 [14]. In particular, rs3918290 and rs55886062 have deleterious effect on DPD activity; whereas rs67376798 and rs75017182 have mild to moderate effect on its activity [15]. Low activity of these enzymes leads to more toxic reactions. rs895819 A/G polymorphism in the DPYD-regulatory microRNA miR-27a is also associated with lower DPD activity [16].

Another well studied anti-cancer drug is Sunitinib, a tyrosine kinase inhibitor [17]. Sunitinib is converted into its active component, N-desethyl metabolite (SU12662) by CYP3A4 [17]. Teo et al. [18] also suggested that the variations in *CYP3A5* may not affect the of the sunitinib metabolism as there is redundancy present between CYP3A5 and CYP3A4 enzymes. Although, CYP3A4 has better affinity towards sunitinib as compared with CYP3A5 [19]. In a Caucasian population, it was observed that the CYP3A4*22 polymorphism is crucial in clearance of sunitinib [20]. However, this polymorphism is not important in Asian population. There are various reports suggesting that these polymorphisms and genetic variations and their outcome vary within different populations so it can be implied that pharmacogenomics is a better approach as compared to pharmacogenetics.

In this chapter, we have tried to elucidate the importance of genetics in the drug therapy. The two important streams of pharmacological sciences: pharmacogenomics and pharmacogenetics, provide important insights into the personalized medicine. Their workflow includes the right drug selection, identification of optimal drug dosing, increasing the efficacy and minimization of drug toxicity. With advancement of basic research, there are better opportunities for the designing 'personalized' gene panels based on genetic and/or genomic profiles to improve the treatment for an individual. However, the integration and implementation of these panels into routine clinical practice remains a major multidisciplinary challenge. Here, we emphasize role of policy makers in incorporation of pharmacogenetics and pharmacogenomics into mainstream clinical practice to improve the drug therapy.

## Author details

Anupam Mittal[1] and Madhu Khullar[2]*

1 Department of Translational and Regenerative Medicine, PGIMER, Chandigarh, India

2 Department of Experimental Medicine and Biotechnology, PGIMER, Chandigarh, India

*Address all correspondence to: madhu.khullar@gmail.com

## References

[1] Food and Drug Administration, HHS. International conference on harmonisation; guidance on E15 pharmacogenomics definitions and sample coding; availability. Notice. Federal Register. 2008;**73**(68):19074-19076

[2] Roden DM, McLeod HL, Relling MV, Williams MS, Mensah GA, Peterson JF, et al. Pharmacogenomics. Lancet London England. 2019;**394**(10197):521-532

[3] Pritchard D, Patel JN, Stephens LE, McLeod HL. Comparison of FDA table of pharmacogenetic associations and clinical pharmacogenetics implementation consortium guidelines. American Journal of Health-System Pharmacy AJHP. 2022;**79**(12):993-1005

[4] Pharm GKB [Internet]. Pharm GKB. Available from: https://www.pharmgkb.org/ [Accessed: January 4, 2024]

[5] Duarte JD, Cavallari LH. Pharmacogenetics to guide cardiovascular drug therapy. Nature Reviews. Cardiology. 2021;**18**(9):649-665

[6] Hopewell JC, Offer A, Haynes R, Bowman L, Li J, Chen F, et al. Independent risk factors for simvastatin-related myopathy and relevance to different types of muscle symptom. European Heart Journal. 2020;**41**(35):3336-3342

[7] Parvez B, Chopra N, Rowan S, Vaglio JC, Muhammad R, Roden DM, et al. A common β1-adrenergic receptor polymorphism predicts favorable response to rate control therapy in atrial fibrillation. Journal of the American College of Cardiology. 2012;**59**(1):49-56

[8] Rysz J, Franczyk B, Rysz-Górzyńska M, Gluba-Brzózka A. Pharmacogenomics of hypertension treatment. International Journal of Molecular Sciences. 2020;**21**(13):4709

[9] Jukic M, Milosavljević F, Molden E, Ingelman-Sundberg M. Pharmacogenomics in treatment of depression and psychosis: An update. Trends in Pharmacological Sciences. 2022;**43**(12):1055-1069

[10] Milosavljevic F, Bukvic N, Pavlovic Z, Miljevic C, Pešic V, Molden E, et al. Association of CYP2C19 and CYP2D6 poor and intermediate metabolizer status with antidepressant and antipsychotic exposure: A systematic review and meta-analysis. JAMA Psychiatry. 2021;**78**(3):270-280

[11] Spear BB, Heath-Chiozzi M, Huff J. Clinical application of pharmacogenetics. Trends in Molecular Medicine. 2001;**7**(5):201-204

[12] Li J, Bluth MH. Pharmacogenomics of drug metabolizing enzymes and transporters: Implications for cancer therapy. Pharmacogenomics and Personalized Medicine. 2011;**4**:11

[13] Aboul-Soud MAM, Alzahrani AJ, Mahmoud A. Decoding variants in drug-metabolizing enzymes and transporters in solid tumor patients by whole-exome sequencing. Saudi Journal of Biological Sciences. 2021;**28**(1):628

[14] Amstutz U, Henricks LM, Offer SM, Barbarino J, Schellens JHM, Swen JJ, et al. Clinical pharmacogenetics implementation consortium (CPIC) guideline for dihydropyrimidine dehydrogenase genotype and fluoropyrimidine dosing: 2017 update. Clinical Pharmacology and Therapeutics. 2018;**103**(2):210-216

[15] Salonga D, Danenberg KD, Johnson M, Metzger R, Groshen S, Tsao-Wei DD, et al. Colorectal tumors responding to 5-fluorouracil have low gene expression levels of dihydropyrimidine dehydrogenase, thymidylate synthase, and thymidine phosphorylase. Clinical Cancer Research. 2000;**6**(4):1322-1327

[16] Offer SM, Butterfield GL, Jerde CR, Fossum CC, Wegner NJ, Diasio RB. MicroRNAs miR-27a and miR-27b directly regulate liver dihydropyrimidine dehydrogenase expression through two conserved binding sites. Molecular Cancer Therapeutics. 2014;**13**(3):742-751

[17] Diekstra MH, Fritsch A, Kanefendt F, Swen JJ, Moes D, Sörgel F, et al. Population modeling integrating pharmacokinetics, pharmacodynamics, pharmacogenetics, and clinical outcome in patients with sunitinib-treated cancer. CPT: Pharmacometrics & Systems Pharmacology. 2017;**6**(9):604-613

[18] Teo YL, Wee HL, Chue XP, Chau NM, Tan MH, Kanesvaran R, et al. Effect of the CYP3A5 and ABCB1 genotype on exposure, clinical response and manifestation of toxicities from sunitinib in Asian patients. The Pharmacogenomics Journal. 2016;**16**(1):47-53

[19] Sugiyama M, Fujita K-i, Murayama N, Akiyama Y, Yamazaki H, Sasaki Y. Sorafenib and sunitinib, two anticancer drugs, inhibit CYP3A4-mediated and activate CY3A5-mediated midazolam 1′-hydroxylation. Drug Metabolism and Disposition. 2011;**39**(5):757-762

[20] Diekstra MHM, Swen JJ, Boven E, Castellano D, Gelderblom H, Mathijssen RHJ, et al. CYP3A5 and ABCB1 polymorphisms as predictors for sunitinib outcome in metastatic renal cell carcinoma. European Urology. 2015;**68**(4):621-629

Chapter 2

# Pharmacogenetics and Pharmacogenomics Impact on Aspirin Response

*Mohd Aftab Siddiqui, Charul Jain, Afreen Usmani, Abdul Hafeez, Mohammad Khalid and Mohd Mujahid*

## Abstract

Aspirin, or Acetylsalicylic acid (ASA), is renowned for its pain-relieving and anti-inflammatory properties. Recent insights have illuminated its mechanisms and potential applications. Notably, low-dose aspirin reduces heart attack and stroke risks, particularly in high-risk individuals, yet optimal dosing remains under investigation. Another area explores aspirin's potential in cancer prevention, especially for colon and gastrointestinal cancers, along with emerging roles against conditions like Alzheimer's, diabetes, and pre-eclampsia. Aspirin's benefits extend to kidney disease and COVID-19 research due to its anti-inflammatory actions. Stem cell effects are diverse; while enhancing hematopoietic stem cells aids bone marrow transplants, it may inhibit embryonic stem cells in specific contexts. However, challenges encompass resistance, allergies, gastrointestinal effects, and pediatric Reye's syndrome. Pharmacogenetic studies illuminate how genetic variations impact aspirin metabolism, with enzymes like CYP2C9 and CYP2C19 affecting clearance rates, and markers such as P2RY12 and COX-1 influencing antiplatelet responses. Customized aspirin therapy, guided by genetic profiles, optimizes benefits and minimizes risks. This research underpins personalized medicine, empowering clinicians to enhance treatment precision, efficacy, and safety. As aspirin's complex advantages and challenges continue to unfold, refined therapeutic strategies will emerge.

**Keywords:** aspirin, acetylsalicylic acid, Pharmacogenetic, anti-inflammatory, analgesic, COVID-19 treatment, cardioprotective effect, neuroprotective effect, stem cell therapy, pre-eclampsia, aspirin resistance, Reye's syndrome

## 1. Introduction

Aspirin, scientifically known as Acetylsalicylic acid (ASA), is a widely used drug that serves multiple purposes, including pain relief, inflammation reduction, and blood clot risk reduction. As a Nonsteroidal anti-inflammatory drug (NSAID), Aspirin (**Figure 1**) works by inhibiting the production of specific molecules

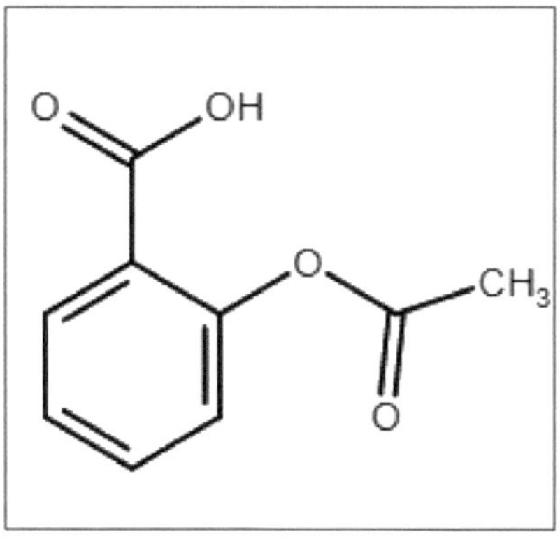

**Figure 1.**
*Chemical structure of aspirin.*

responsible for pain and inflammation. It finds extensive use in treating various conditions, such as menstrual cramps, toothaches, headaches, and fever [1].

The history of aspirin dates back to ancient civilizations, with ancient Sumerians and Egyptians using willow bark and leaves to address inflammatory diseases and alleviate joint pain. Hippocrates, the father of medicine, recommended using Cortex salicis for labor pain and ocular pain. In 1828, Professor Johann Buchner discovered salicin, a yellow bitter crystal extracted from willow bark, which was later converted to salicylic acid (SA) through various chemical processes. In 1838, the French chemist Charles Frederich Gerhardt successfully acetylated salicylic acid, producing ASA for the first time. However, it was only in 1899 that Bayer & Co. made ASA available in powder form, registering it under the name "Aspirin." Today, aspirin is a widely recognized and essential medication, with an estimated annual consumption of 44,000 tonnes (50–120 billion pills), and it is listed on the World Health Organization's list of essential medicines [2, 3].

Aspirin is available in various doses and forms, including chewable tablets, suppositories, and extended-release formulations. The two primary forms are enteric-coated and immediate-release aspirin. Immediate-release aspirin is quickly and completely absorbed after oral intake in the acidic conditions of the stomach and upper small intestine, resulting in a quick peak concentration. In contrast, enteric-coated aspirin is absorbed by the gastrointestinal mucosa due to the elevated pH in the small intestine, leading to a reduced bioavailability and slower peak concentration. Salicylate, the active component of aspirin, primarily binds to albumin in the blood and is mainly excreted through the kidneys as salicyluric acid. In cases of aspirin overdose, urinary alkalinization is used to promote salicylate elimination, as renal excretion of salicylic acid is sensitive to variations in urinary pH [4, 5].

Aspirin acts on its targets in the portal circulation, where platelets are exposed to a higher drug level than in the systemic circulation. Up to 80% of therapeutic doses of aspirin are metabolized (deactivated) in the liver. Although aspirin has a short half-life of 15 to 20 minutes, its pharmacodynamic effects on platelets last for the entire lifespan of platelets, which is approximately 7 to 10 days. This effect can only be countered by generating new platelets, although there are suggestions that ASA may have inhibitory effects on blood marrow megakaryocytes [6].

The irreversible acetylation of platelets by ASA can be inhibited by concurrent use of reversible COX-1 inhibitors, such as ibuprofen and naproxen, leading to a reduction in aspirin's antiplatelet effects. Additionally, coadministering non-selective NSAIDs with aspirin can increase the risk of thrombotic and bleeding events [7, 8].

Aspirin's primary application lies in preventing cardiovascular and cerebrovascular diseases, particularly in reducing the risk of heart attacks and strokes. It achieves this by inhibiting the function of thromboxane A2, which helps minimize the formation of blood clots [9, 10]. Aspirin's effects, such as inflammation reduction, analgesia, clotting prevention, and fever reduction, are largely attributed to its impact on prostaglandin and thromboxane production, both derived from arachidonic acid. As the only NSAID capable of covalently acetylating and irreversibly inactivating both COX-1 and COX-2 enzyme isoforms, aspirin exhibits a unique pharmacological profile. COX-1 inhibition mainly leads to an antiplatelet effect, while COX-2 inhibition provides anti-inflammatory effects [11, 12].

The mechanism of action of aspirin involves irreversible acetylation of platelets, which inhibits cyclooxygenase (COX) enzymes, specifically COX-1 and COX-2. COX-1 inhibition mainly contributes to its antiplatelet effect, while COX-2 inhibition provides anti-inflammatory effects [13]. This property makes aspirin unique among NSAIDs. Its short half-life of 15 to 20 minutes belies its prolonged pharmacodynamic effects on platelets that last for the entire platelet lifespan (7 to 10 days) [14]. Because nucleated cells quickly resynthesize the enzyme, pathophysiologic processes that depend on COX-2 need for higher doses and a shorter dosing interval [15]. Reduced platelet aggregation can be achieved with low-dose ASA (75–80 mg). However, for anti-inflammatory activity, a greater dose (>325 mg) is required [16, 17].

Due to the substantial variability in individual responses to aspirin therapy, there is significant interest in exploring the pharmacogenetic and pharmacogenomic aspects of aspirin treatment. Pharmacogenetics and pharmacogenomics are fields that study how genetic variations influence drug metabolism, transport, and target interactions. These disciplines offer valuable insights into individual variations in drug efficacy, safety, and adverse reactions, paving the way for personalized medicine approaches in drug therapy [18].

The metabolism and bioactivation of aspirin are crucial factors in understanding its pharmacogenetic profile. Hepatic metabolism through ester hydrolysis leads to the formation of salicylic acid, the active metabolite responsible for aspirin's therapeutic effects. Genetic polymorphisms in the CYP2C9 gene, a member of the cytochrome P450 family, significantly impact aspirin's metabolism, leading to variations in drug levels and platelet inhibition. Patients with specific CYP2C9 variants may experience altered drug clearance, resulting in either reduced or enhanced platelet inhibition, with implications for the clinical response to aspirin therapy [19].

In addition to metabolism, the pharmacogenetic aspect of aspirin therapy also involves variations in the target receptor, cyclooxygenase (COX). Aspirin's antiplatelet effects are mediated through the irreversible acetylation of a serine residue in the COX-1 enzyme, inhibiting its activity and preventing the production of thromboxane A2. Genetic variations in the COX-1 gene may influence the enzyme's activity and alter the degree of platelet inhibition achieved with aspirin therapy. For instance, certain genetic variants have been associated with reduced COX-1 activity, potentially leading to suboptimal antiplatelet effects of aspirin in some individuals [20].

Furthermore, the emerging field of pharmacogenomics has provided new avenues to explore the genetic determinants of aspirin drug therapy. Genome-wide association studies (GWAS) have identified genetic loci associated with aspirin response, shedding light on novel pathways and biological processes that influence aspirin's pharmacodynamics and pharmacokinetics. Pharmacogenomic investigations have uncovered gene-gene and gene-environment interactions that may impact aspirin therapy outcomes. These findings not only offer insights into aspirin's individual variability but also pave the way for the development of more targeted and effective treatment approaches [21].

Understanding the genetic factors that influence aspirin metabolism and response can lead to more personalized and effective drug therapies, advancing the future of precision medicine in healthcare. In this chapter challenges, applications, Pharmacogenomics & Pharmacogenetics aspects related to aspirin are discussed.

## 2. Challenges in aspirin therapy

### 2.1 Aspirin sensitivity

Aspirin sensitivity, also known as an aspirin-related adverse event, can lead to various symptoms, including nasal congestion, runny nose, hives, and breathing difficulties. In severe cases, it may even cause anaphylaxis, a life-threatening allergic reaction [22]. There are two main mechanisms for aspirin sensitivity: non-immunologic reactions, primarily involving the inhibition of the cyclooxygenase (COX)-1 pathway, and immunological responses, which often require drug-specific IgE generation against the NSAID. Immunological reactions can lead to urticaria/angioedema and, in rare instances, anaphylaxis, while COX-1 inhibition by aspirin can cause respiratory issues [23].

To address aspirin sensitivity, desensitization therapy is commonly employed. The goal of desensitization is to reduce or eliminate adverse reactions when taking aspirin. This process involves starting with a small dose and gradually increasing it over time to help the individual's body develop tolerance to the medication. It's important to note that desensitization is not a cure, and some individuals may not respond well to it. People with aspirin-exacerbated respiratory disease (AERD), which involves asthma, nasal polyps, and aspirin sensitivity, as well as those with urticaria and Kawasaki disease, have been found to benefit from aspirin desensitization [24].

### 2.2 Aspirin resistance

Aspirin resistance refers to the failure of aspirin to decrease thromboxane A2 synthesis by platelets, leading to platelet activation and aggregation. This condition can be caused by various factors such as genetics, obesity, and specific medical disorders. Aspirin resistance may increase the risk of heart attack, stroke, and other thrombotic events. Laboratory tests are used to identify aspirin resistance by measuring platelet thromboxane A2 production or platelet function that relies on platelet thromboxane production. The underlying causes of aspirin resistance may include insufficient dosage, medication interactions, genetic polymorphisms in COX-1 and other thromboxane biosynthesis-related genes, overexpression of non-platelet sources of thromboxane production, and accelerated platelet turnover. Addressing the underlying cause can help reverse aspirin resistance. Research is ongoing to better understand this phenomenon and develop accurate diagnostics and potential treatments [25, 26].

### 2.3 Gastrointestinal problems

Aspirin is rapidly absorbed in the proximal small intestine and stomach. Factors such as the amount of fluid ingested with aspirin, the pH of the gastrointestinal tract, rate of gastric emptying, presence of food, and the type of aspirin formulation can affect its absorption. Taking aspirin after eating is recommended to reduce gastrotoxicity, but it may impact its bioavailability and efficacy. The acidic nature of aspirin can lead to passive diffusion and trapping in the gastric mucosal cell, causing gastrotoxicity. Additionally, aspirin inhibits the gastroprotective effects of PGE2 and PGI2 by inhibiting COX-1 in the stomach. Gastrointestinal complications, such as ulcers and bleeding, are more likely when taking higher or lower than 100 mg of aspirin daily [27–30].

To minimize gastrotoxicity while enhancing bioavailability, various methods of administering aspirin have been suggested. These include using a diluted acetylsalicylate solution, an intravenous injection solution, a quickly dissolving tablet, a solution with added antacid, a fine-grained, highly buffered aspirin tablet, an enteric-coated tablet, or an aspirin substitute like acetaminophen [31, 32].

### 2.4 Reye syndrome

Reye syndrome is a rare and potentially fatal pediatric disease characterized by acute non-inflammatory encephalopathy with fatty liver failure. Epidemiological studies have shown a connection between Reye syndrome and the consumption of aspirin during or after a viral infection. Aspirin's damage to cellular mitochondria may inhibit fatty-acid metabolism, leading to hepatic mitochondrial failure and high ammonia levels, which contribute to the neurologic symptoms of Reye syndrome. Reye syndrome cases significantly decreased after public cautions were issued against administering aspirin to children in the 1980s [33–35].

### 2.5 Aspirin withdrawal syndromes

Abruptly stopping aspirin, like many other medications, can lead to withdrawal syndromes, and in some cases, it can be fatal. The discontinuation of aspirin may transiently increase the risk of thrombotic events. Research has shown that aspirin withdrawal can cause a prothrombotic state in both clinical and animal studies. Some studies suggest that patients with known coronary disease may face a higher risk of new coronary events if they stop taking aspirin. Hence, it is crucial to identify at-risk individuals and inform them about the risks associated with aspirin discontinuation [36–38].

## 3. Unraveling Aspirin's expanded applications

### 3.1 Aspirin in myocardial infarction

Cardiovascular disease, mainly caused by severe atherosclerosis, often leads to myocardial infarction due to thrombotic blockage of major coronary arteries. The primary cause of thrombus formation is the rupture of atherosclerotic plaques [39]. Aspirin is the preferred drug for long-term prevention of secondary myocardial infarction and stroke.

Current guidelines recommend a daily dose of 75 mg according to the ESC Guidelines, while other recommendations range between 100 and 150 mg. The use of aspirin for secondary prevention lowers the risk of new vascular events by about 20–25% overall [40, 41].

For males aged 45 to 70, aspirin is recommended for preventive measures if the potential benefit of reducing the risk of myocardial infarction outweighs the potential risk of bleeding (gastrointestinal or cerebral hemorrhage). Similarly, women aged 55 to 79 are advised to take aspirin for prophylaxis if the risk of ischemic stroke is reduced more than the potential risk of bleeding. In the US guidelines, the prescription for long-term cardiovascular protection ranges from 75 to 325 mg/day and tends to decrease over time [42].

Antiplatelet agents, particularly aspirin, play a crucial role in treating acute coronary syndromes by preventing existing thrombi from growing and new ones from forming. One significant trial, the ISIS-2 trial, highlighted the clinical significance of aspirin in acute myocardial infarction, both as monotherapy and in combination with thrombolysis to reopen occluded coronary arteries [43].

### 3.2 Aspirin in cerebrovascular events (stroke)

Cerebral ischemia, caused by obstructions in cerebral circulation, leads to decreased cerebral blood flow [44]. This condition can manifest as transient ischemic attacks (TIAs) or reversible and irreversible disabling strokes. Studies have investigated the use of high-dose intravenous aspirin (500 mg) in reducing cerebral microemboli in patients with recent strokes of arterial origin [45].

Various aspirin dosages may be needed to inhibit platelet aggregation and thrombogenesis caused by different platelet activation triggers [46]. Clinical data on the outcomes of different aspirin dosages in stroke patients are not yet fully outlined. Two significant clinical trials, the Dutch TIA study and the UK TIA trial, showed no difference in outcomes between low doses (30 mg/day and 283 mg/day) and larger doses (300 mg versus 1200 mg daily), although the larger doses resulted in more hemorrhage [47, 48].

The US guidelines recommend 325 mg of oral aspirin within the first 24 to 48 hours following the onset of a stroke [49].

Aspirin's importance in stroke patients is further highlighted by the recurrence of thrombotic cerebrovascular events after aspirin is removed, underscoring the significance of aspirin-induced platelet activity restriction for clinical prognosis [50–53].

### 3.3 Aspirin in peripheral arterial occlusive disease (PAD)

Peripheral arterial occlusive disease (PAD) is characterized by peripheral artery stenosis and occlusion, with the lower limbs being most commonly affected [54, 55].

Aspirin has been extensively studied as an antiplatelet medication for PAD. However, aspirin-resistant platelets are common in PAD patients [56–66].

For all PAD patients, it is recommended to evaluate other authorized antiplatelet medications and consider combining aspirin with medications to lower blood pressure and cholesterol, as well as encouraging smoking cessation for optimal clinical impact [67].

### 3.4 Aspirin in venous thromboembolism (VTE)

Venous thromboembolism (VTE) is a serious and potentially fatal side effect of acute surgical procedures, usually presenting as deep vein thrombosis (DVT) with pulmonary embolism (PE) as the main complication [68].

Aspirin influences various targets to alter the production of venous thrombus, primarily by preventing the synthesis of thromboxane and reducing thrombin production, thus reducing platelet aggregation at antiplatelet dosages [69–71].

Studies like the "Warfarin and Acetylsalicylic Acid" (WARFASA) research and the "Aspirin to Prevent Recurrent Venous Thromboembolism" (ASPIRE) study have explored whether low-dose aspirin can be effective in preventing VTE after guideline-directed anticoagulation [72, 73].

### 3.5 Preeclampsia

Preeclampsia is a major risk factor for preterm birth and a leading cause of maternal and fetal mortality. It is characterized by hypertension, proteinuria, and a severe maternal systemic inflammatory response [74, 75]. Insufficient production of prostacyclin (PGI2) during early gestation is linked to the pathophysiology of pregnancy-induced hypertension (PIH). Aspirin, due to its anti-inflammatory and anticoagulant properties, is suggested as a possible effective treatment option for Preeclampsia [76–83]. Aspirin's ability to cross the placenta and work at 50–150 mg makes it a useful therapy, but >75 mg/day is better [84].

The American College of Obstetrics and Gynecology and the Society for Maternal-Fetal Medicine recommend starting low-dose aspirin (81 mg/day) between 12 and 28 weeks of pregnancy for PE prevention, continuing daily until delivery for women at high risk of PE. Low-dose aspirin during early pregnancy is generally safe for the fetus and newborn [85, 86].

Aspirin appears safe for preterm prelabour membrane rupture. Its efficacy in reducing preterm rupture risk is uncertain [87]. Finding a safe and effective dose for women with medical conditions remains a priority, as certain disorders may reduce aspirin's effectiveness [88, 89].

### 3.6 Cancer prevention

Inflammation plays a role in various diseases, including cancer. ASA shows promise as a chemo-preventive drug against colorectal, breast, lung, stomach, ovarian, hepatic, and prostate cancers. ASA's mechanisms involve inhibiting COX-2, elevating arachidonic acid, and influencing sphingosine pathways. Low doses of ASA are effective in breast and colon cancer prevention. ASA's impact on Wnt/b-catenin pathway and NF-B activation further supports its anti-cancer potential. Regular aspirin use is associated with lower colorectal cancer incidence and mortality rates. It may also benefit patients with breast and prostate cancer. Daily antiplatelet doses of 75–100 mg appear effective in preventing tumor recurrence and suppressing metastases. However, aspirin's role in primary cancer prevention and individual tumor response requires further investigation, considering both benefits and risks [16, 90–110].

### 3.7 Neurological disorders

Neuropsychiatric disorders, including Alzheimer's disease, affect the central nervous system and are characterized by protein buildup and synaptic dysfunction [111]. The pathogenesis involves neuroinflammation and mitochondrial dysfunction [112, 113]. β-amyloid leads to mitochondrial dysfunction and inflammation, making neurons more susceptible to ischemia responses [113]. Prolonged neuroinflammation may contribute to β-amyloid accumulation in plaques, and platelets are a significant source of β-amyloid, suggesting APP as an Alzheimer's biomarker [114–117]. Cognitive deficits in Alzheimer's patients are related to β-amyloid oligomers in the CNS [118]. Aspirin has shown potential in reducing amyloid aggregates and inflammation [119–121]. However, existing therapies have not yielded definitive results due to the complexity of the disease [122, 123]. Aspirin's anti-thrombotic properties may help prevent cognitive decline caused by ischemia and it could target apolipoprotein E isoforms and inflammatory substances [124]. Epidemiological trials suggest that NSAIDs, including aspirin, when taken early and consistently for two or more years, may lower the prevalence of Alzheimer's. Nevertheless, to confirm these findings, more comprehensive, large-scale, prospective randomized studies considering genetic variants and risk factors are needed. Presently, there are no substantial prospective trials on aspirin for Alzheimer's prevention or treatment [125].

### 3.8 Role of aspirin in COVID-19

COVID-19 is associated with an increased risk of thrombosis, and aspirin has been shown to reduce platelet activation in COVID-19 patients. Anticoagulation and aspirin have been recommended for severe COVID-19 patients [126–131]. Anticoagulant treatment reduced mortality in severe COVID-19 patients [132]. Aspirin decreased platelet activation in COVID-19 patients, while studies showed increased platelet reactivity inhibited by high-dose aspirin in vitro [133–136]. Autopsies revealed high rates of thromboembolic incidents, highlighting COVID-19-induced coagulopathy and the need for further research on potential therapeutic approaches [137]. Aspirin may have potential antiviral effects, but more research is needed in this area [138–140].

### 3.9 Effect of aspirin in renal disease

Limited research exists on low-dose aspirin regimens (75 to 325 mg/d). A recent finding indicates that 75 mg of aspirin reduces uric acid and creatinine excretion in older patients [141, 142]. In most cases, except for patients with renal insufficiency, cirrhosis, or heart failure, aspirin does not affect renal function when taken in anti-inflammatory doses [143–145].

### 3.10 Impact of aspirin in stem cell therapy

Aspirin has been found to have positive effects on various stem cell functions and therapies. In preclinical studies, aspirin has been shown to enhance the functions of different stem cell types. For example, it promotes the functions of osteogenic, tenogenic, and cardiomyocyte stem cells. Co-treatment of aspirin with stem cells has also been found to enhance their immunomodulatory capabilities [146].

Studies have shown that aspirin exposure affects stem cell behavior in both in vitro and in vivo environments. The duration and dosage of aspirin exposure determine the extent to which it influences stem cell growth and functions. For instance, aspirin has been shown to induce the death of mesenchymal stem cells via the Wnt/catenin pathway [147].

In treating bone abnormalities, aspirin treatment has been found to improve bone repair caused by bone marrow mesenchymal stem cells [148]. In other studies, aspirin has been demonstrated to enhance the osteogenic potential of human dental pulp stem cells and human mesenchymal stem cells [149, 150].

### 3.11 Kawasaki's disease

Kawasaki's disease is a pediatric vasculitis characterized by various clinical manifestations, such as high fever, rashes, and cervical lymphadenopathy. Aspirin has been used in the treatment of Kawasaki's disease, typically in conjunction with intravenous immunoglobulin (IVIG). During the acute stage of the disease, high-dose aspirin is administered at anti-inflammatory levels (80 to 100 mg/kg per day) along with IVIG [151, 152].

The use of aspirin during the acute stage of Kawasaki's disease has been found to reduce fever duration and lower hemoglobin levels [153]. Following the acute phase, low-dose aspirin is continued for six to eight weeks to reduce the risk of coronary artery aneurysms [154]. A meta-analysis on the effectiveness of aspirin in Kawasaki's disease revealed that the risk of coronary artery aneurysms is reduced by 9% and 4% when high-dose aspirin is administered along with IVIG within 30 and 60 days of disease onset, respectively [155].

## 4. Genetic influence on aspirin response: exploring through pharmacogenetics and pharmacogenomics

Pharmacogenetics, the study of how genetic variations influence drug responses, has emerged as a groundbreaking field in medicine. It provides valuable insights into individual variations in drug metabolism, efficacy, and safety, offering the promise of personalized therapies. Aspirin, a widely used medication known for its antiplatelet effects in cardiovascular disease prevention, is one such drug whose efficacy can be influenced by genetic factors. This article explores the role of pharmacogenetics in understanding genetic variants affecting aspirin response, with a focus on the impact of COX-1 gene polymorphisms, drug metabolizing enzyme variants (e.g., CYP2C19), and genetic variability in platelet receptors and pathways.

### 4.1 COX-1 gene polymorphisms and aspirin resistance

The COX-1 gene contains the genetic instructions needed to produce an enzyme called cyclooxygenase-1. This enzyme plays a critical role in the creation of molecules called prostaglandins. Prostaglandins are involved in various physiological processes, including promoting inflammation, contributing to pain signaling, and participating in the formation of blood clots. Aspirin functions by irreversibly inhibiting COX-1, preventing its normal activity. This inhibition leads to a decrease in the production of prostaglandins, which in turn reduces inflammation and pain, as well as lowers the likelihood of blood clot formation.

Despite aspirin's effectiveness, some individuals might not experience the anticipated results from its use. This condition is known as aspirin resistance. In cases of aspirin resistance, the expected outcomes, such as reduced blood clot formation, might not be achieved as effectively.

Aspirin resistance can be attributed to genetic variations within the COX-1 gene. These genetic differences can result in alterations in the structure and function of the COX-1 enzyme. One well-known genetic alteration is called the A-842G polymorphism, also referred to as C50T or rs3842787 SNP. This particular genetic variant has gained recognition due to its association with a diminished suppression of COX-1 activity by aspirin. Consequently, the ability of aspirin to prevent platelet aggregation, a key step in clot formation, is compromised in individuals carrying this genetic variant.

The implications of possessing the A-842G polymorphism are notable. Individuals with this genetic variation might face an increased risk of cardiovascular incidents, even when undergoing aspirin therapy. This elevated risk is attributed to the reduced effectiveness of aspirin in preventing platelet aggregation, which can contribute to the formation of blood clots and subsequent cardiovascular events [156].

### 4.2 Genetic variability in CYP2C19 enzyme and its impact on aspirin metabolism

Aspirin is transformed within the liver through a series of biochemical processes, involving various enzymes responsible for breaking down the drug. Among these enzymes, the cytochrome P450 (CYP) enzymes play a primary role. However, genetic differences in these enzymes can have a significant impact on how aspirin is processed, which can result in varying levels of its effectiveness and safety.

An essential enzyme in the metabolism of aspirin is known as CYP2C19. This enzyme is responsible for converting aspirin into its active form through a chemical reaction. However, genetic variations, or polymorphisms, occurring within the CYP2C19 gene can lead to reduced activity of this enzyme. This reduction in enzyme activity directly affects the speed and efficiency with which aspirin is converted into its active form.

Individuals who carry genetic variants that result in poor CYP2C19 metabolism might experience a diminished response to aspirin treatment. Essentially, their bodies might not process aspirin as effectively, which could lead to a weaker impact in terms of its intended effects.

The consequences of this genetic variability can be clinically significant, particularly in the context of cardiovascular health. Reduced responsiveness to aspirin therapy due to poor CYP2C19 metabolizer status has been associated with an increased risk of experiencing negative cardiovascular events. In simpler terms, individuals with certain genetic variants might not receive the expected benefits from aspirin, and this could potentially lead to more adverse outcomes related to heart health [157].

### 4.3 P2Y12 receptor gene variation and aspirin response

Aspirin exerts its ability to prevent blood clot formation primarily by inhibiting an enzyme called COX-1. However, beyond this mechanism, there are genetic factors that influence the way platelet receptors and pathways respond to aspirin's effects.

One such example involves a genetic variation known as rs5918, found within the gene responsible for producing the P2Y12 receptor. The P2Y12 receptor plays a significant role in the activation and aggregation of platelets, which are essential steps in the clotting process. Depending on an individual's genetic makeup, specifically the alleles they carry for this variation, such as the C34T allele, their response to aspirin can be affected. Studies have revealed that individuals with certain variants of rs5918 might experience reduced platelet inhibition when exposed to aspirin. This diminished response can potentially weaken aspirin's effectiveness in preventing the formation of blood clots.

Moreover, genetic variability in other platelet pathways also plays a role in influencing how aspirin's effects are modulated. For instance, pathways involving the glycoprotein IIb/IIIa receptor, another crucial player in platelet activation, can be influenced by genetic differences. These variations can lead to differences in how aspirin interacts with these receptors and pathways, potentially impacting its ability to inhibit platelet aggregation effectively [158].

In essence, while aspirin's primary action is mediated through COX-1 inhibition, genetic factors related to platelet receptors and pathways contribute to the overall response to aspirin therapy. Variations in genes like rs5918 and pathways involving receptors like glycoprotein IIb/IIIa can impact an individual's platelet response to aspirin. This underscores the complexity of how genetics can influence drug interactions and responses, and highlights the importance of considering genetic factors when tailoring treatment plans for optimal patient outcomes.

### 4.4 Impact of SLCO1B1 gene variants on aspirin absorption and metabolism

The SLCO1B1 gene is a crucial player in the absorption and metabolism of various drugs, including aspirin, by encoding a protein responsible for transporting these substances into liver cells. This gene is a member of the organic anion transporting polypeptide (OATP) family, which facilitates the uptake of a wide range of compounds into hepatocytes (liver cells). Variants or mutations in the SLCO1B1 gene can influence its functionality, leading to alterations in drug absorption, distribution, metabolism, and excretion (ADME) processes.

The liver plays a central role in drug metabolism, as it processes drugs to make them more water-soluble and easier to eliminate from the body. The SLCO1B1 protein contributes to this process by transporting drugs and their metabolites from the bloodstream into the liver cells, where they can undergo further metabolic transformations.

Several studies have investigated the impact of SLCO1B1 gene variants on drug response and adverse reactions. One well-studied example is the influence of SLCO1B1 variants on statin medications, which are commonly prescribed to lower cholesterol levels. Some specific SLCO1B1 variants have been associated with decreased transport of certain statins into the liver cells, resulting in higher systemic drug concentrations. This can increase the risk of side effects, particularly muscle-related adverse events.

In the context of aspirin, variations in the SLCO1B1 gene may affect the liver's ability to absorb and metabolize the drug. Aspirin is a widely used nonsteroidal anti-inflammatory drug (NSAID) that also has antiplatelet effects, making it valuable for preventing cardiovascular events. However, genetic differences in drug metabolism can lead to variability in aspirin's efficacy and safety.

The concept of pharmacogenetics explores how individual genetic makeup influences responses to drugs. Understanding the impact of specific genetic variants on drug handling can help tailor medication regimens for patients, optimizing therapeutic outcomes while minimizing adverse effects. In the case of SLCO1B1 gene variants, genetic testing could offer insights into an individual's ability to metabolize and respond to drugs like aspirin.

It's important to note that while the SLCO1B1 gene's significance in drug transport and metabolism is well-established, individual responses to drugs are influenced by a complex interplay of genetic, environmental, and physiological factors. Genetic testing and personalized medicine are rapidly evolving fields that aim to provide more precise and effective treatment strategies [159–162].

### 4.5 Genetic variations in ABCB1 gene and Aspirin's antiplatelet effects

The ABCB1 gene, also known as the multidrug resistance 1 (MDR1) gene, encodes a protein called P-glycoprotein (P-gp) that functions as an efflux transporter. P-gp is widely expressed in various tissues, including the intestines, liver, and blood-brain barrier. Its primary role is to transport a diverse range of substances, including drugs, toxins, and metabolites, out of cells. In the context of drug therapy, P-gp plays a crucial role in regulating the absorption and distribution of drugs, thereby affecting their bioavailability and efficacy.

The transport activity of P-gp is particularly important in cells that line blood vessels and in organs like the kidneys. In blood vessel lining cells, P-gp helps in transporting drugs from these cells back into the bloodstream, limiting their accumulation within the cells. This mechanism can affect the overall distribution and clearance of drugs, influencing their therapeutic effects and potential side effects.

Aspirin, an NSAID with anti-inflammatory and antiplatelet effects, is one of the drugs influenced by genetic variations in the ABCB1 gene. Aspirin is widely used for its antiplatelet properties, which help prevent blood clot formation and reduce the risk of cardiovascular events. The ability of aspirin to exit cells, including platelets, is influenced by P-gp-mediated transport. Genetic differences in the ABCB1 gene can lead to variations in P-gp activity, which in turn affects aspirin's movement out of cells and its overall antiplatelet effects.

Several studies have explored the impact of ABCB1 gene variants on drug responses and clinical outcomes. Variations in the ABCB1 gene have been associated with altered drug pharmacokinetics, efficacy, and safety profiles. For example, individuals with certain ABCB1 gene variants might have reduced P-gp activity, leading to altered drug distribution and potential differences in treatment response [163–167].

## 4.6 Role of genetic polymorphisms in ITGA2 gene and Aspirin response

The ITGA2 gene encodes a protein known as integrin alpha-2 ($\alpha 2$), which is a platelet receptor involved in the process of platelet aggregation and blood clotting. Integrins are cell adhesion molecules that play a key role in linking cells to the extracellular matrix and other cells, and they are particularly important for platelet function. Platelets are crucial components of blood that play a pivotal role in forming blood clots to prevent excessive bleeding.

The integrin alpha-2$\beta$1 receptor, formed by the combination of integrin alpha-2 and beta-1 subunits, is present on the surface of platelets. It facilitates platelet adhesion to collagen, a component of the extracellular matrix, and is essential for the initial stages of blood clot formation at sites of vascular injury. This adhesion is a critical step in platelet aggregation, which leads to the formation of a stable blood clot that prevents further bleeding.

The effectiveness of aspirin in preventing platelet aggregation and reducing the risk of blood clots may be influenced by genetic variations in the ITGA2 gene. Genetic polymorphisms in this gene could potentially impact the structure and function of the integrin alpha-2 receptor, affecting its ability to interact with collagen and initiate platelet aggregation. Aspirin, a well-known antiplatelet agent, works by inhibiting the production of certain molecules that promote platelet aggregation, thereby reducing the risk of clot formation.

Research has shown that genetic variations in platelet receptors like integrins can influence the responsiveness of platelets to antiplatelet agents, including aspirin. These variations might lead to differences in platelet aggregation, clot formation, and response to aspirin therapy. Therefore, understanding the role of genetic polymorphisms in the ITGA2 gene and their impact on platelet function could provide valuable insights into individual variability in aspirin's antiplatelet effects [168–172].

### 4.7 Potential influence of PGF and TXB2 gene variations on Aspirin's antiplatelet effects

Genetic variations in the genes responsible for the synthesis of prostaglandins (PGF) and thromboxanes (TXB2) can have a significant impact on how aspirin functions as an anti-inflammatory and antiplatelet agent. Aspirin's mechanism of action involves inhibiting the production of prostaglandins and thromboxanes, which are important signaling molecules involved in various physiological processes, including inflammation and platelet aggregation.

Prostaglandins and thromboxanes are derived from arachidonic acid, a fatty acid found in cell membranes. These molecules play critical roles in regulating inflammation, blood vessel dilation and constriction, and platelet activation. Prostaglandins are involved in mediating pain, fever, and inflammation, while thromboxanes contribute to platelet aggregation and blood clot formation.

Aspirin exerts its effects by irreversibly inhibiting the enzyme cyclooxygenase (COX), particularly COX-1 and COX-2. COX enzymes are responsible for converting arachidonic acid into prostaglandins and thromboxanes. By inhibiting COX, aspirin reduces the production of these molecules, which leads to decreased inflammation and inhibited platelet aggregation.

Genetic variations in the genes encoding key enzymes involved in prostaglandin and thromboxane synthesis can influence how aspirin affects these processes. Variants in these genes may lead to altered enzyme activity, resulting in variations in the levels of prostaglandins and thromboxanes even in the presence of aspirin.

Aspirin's anti-inflammatory and antiplatelet effects are crucial for its therapeutic benefits, such as reducing the risk of cardiovascular events. Genetic differences in the PGF and TXB2 genes could potentially impact aspirin's efficacy in suppressing inflammation and platelet activation. This could translate to variability in aspirin's ability to prevent blood clot formation and reduce the risk of adverse cardiovascular events.

Pharmacogenetic studies in this area aim to elucidate the relationship between genetic variations and aspirin response. By identifying genetic markers associated with altered aspirin metabolism or activity, healthcare providers can potentially tailor aspirin dosages or recommend alternative treatments to optimize therapeutic outcomes while minimizing risks [173].

### 4.8 CYP2C9 gene variations as a key factor in aspirin response and bleeding risk

The CYP2C9 gene encodes an enzyme responsible for metabolizing various drugs, including aspirin. Genetic variations within the CYP2C9 gene can impact the rate at which this enzyme metabolizes aspirin, leading to variability in drug metabolism and response. One significant aspect influenced by these genetic differences is the risk of bleeding due to altered aspirin metabolism.

Specific variants of the CYP2C9 gene are associated with reduced enzyme activity, resulting in slower metabolization of aspirin. Consequently, individuals carrying these variants may experience higher levels of aspirin in their bloodstream after taking a standard dose. This elevated drug concentration can potentiate aspirin's antiplatelet effects, increasing the risk of bleeding events. Patients with such genetic variants might be more susceptible to bleeding complications, especially in situations requiring surgery or other interventions.

To mitigate the bleeding risk while maintaining aspirin's therapeutic benefits, personalized dosing strategies can be employed. Lower aspirin doses might be necessary for individuals with reduced CYP2C9 enzyme activity. By aligning the dosage with an individual's genetic makeup, healthcare providers can balance the antiplatelet effects of aspirin with the potential bleeding risk, offering a safer and more effective treatment approach [174, 175].

### 4.9 GPIa polymorphism and aspirin response

The GPIa C807T polymorphism has been the subject of investigation in various studies focusing on both surrogate and clinical outcomes, particularly in patients with coronary artery disease (CAD) who are undergoing aspirin therapy. However, the collective findings from these studies have consistently indicated that the GPIa C807T polymorphism does not significantly contribute to the variability observed in the response to aspirin.

Multiple investigations into surrogate and clinical endpoints have consistently failed to establish a substantial role for the GPIa C807T polymorphism in accounting for the variability in aspirin response among CAD patients. Despite its potential involvement in platelet function and thrombotic processes, this specific genetic variation does not seem to play a significant role in influencing the efficacy of aspirin treatment in these individuals.

In contrast, other genetic factors have been explored in relation to aspirin response. The GPIba C-5 T polymorphism, another genetic variation associated with platelet function, has shown potential significance. Studies have suggested that GPIba C-5 T might contribute to the development of aspirin resistance in patients. This implies that individuals carrying this particular genetic variant may be more likely to exhibit reduced responsiveness to aspirin's antiplatelet effects, which could impact the therapeutic benefits of the treatment.

Furthermore, investigations have also extended to other genetic markers, such as GPIaa C807T and COX-2G-765C. These studies aimed to understand their roles in influencing the response of patients undergoing aspirin therapy. The results have indicated that while GPIaa C807T does not appear to be a significant determinant of aspirin responsiveness, the COX-2G-765C variant also does not appear to significantly contribute to the response variability of patients on aspirin therapy [176].

### 4.10 Impact of GPIIIa polymorphism on aspirin response

The platelet glycoprotein IIIa (GPIIIa) is a component of the GPIIb/IIIa complex, serving as the receptor for fibrinogen and other adhesive molecules. Encoded by the ITGB3 gene, GPIIIa plays a critical role in platelet aggregation. A diallelic polymorphism of the ITGB3 gene, known as the PlA1/A2 polymorphism, affects platelet function. This polymorphism involves a single transition at position 1565 in exon 2 of the gene, resulting in two allelic variants: P1A1 and P1A2.

The GPIIb/IIIa complex, formed by the combination of GPIIb and GPIIIa, is essential for platelet aggregation, an integral step in forming blood clots. Fibrinogen and other adhesive molecules bind to this complex, promoting platelet aggregation at sites of vascular injury. The PlA1/A2 polymorphism influences the structure and function of GPIIIa, potentially impacting platelet aggregation and overall thrombotic processes.

Among individuals of white ethnicity, about 25% express the P1A2 allele, characterized by a Leu 33 Pro substitution. The P1A2 allele has been implicated as a potential risk factor for coronary artery disease (CAD) in some studies, though this association has not been universally confirmed.

In the context of aspirin therapy and CAD, conflicting results have emerged from studies. Research involving patients with stable CAD who received aspirin doses ranging from 80 to 325 mg/day revealed contradictory findings regarding the impact of the PlA1/A2 genotype. Some studies reported an association between the PlA1/A1 genotype and a twofold increased risk of high platelet reactivity, as assessed using the Platelet Function Analyzer-100 (PFA-100).

These results suggest that the PlA1/A2 polymorphism of the ITGB3 gene can influence platelet reactivity and potentially contribute to the variability in aspirin response observed in patients with CAD. The conflicting outcomes underscore the complexity of genetic influences on platelet function and aspirin's antiplatelet effects. The PlA1/A2 polymorphism's role in cardiovascular risk and aspirin responsiveness necessitates further research to fully elucidate its impact and potential clinical implications [177, 178].

## 5. Clinical implications of genetic testing for aspirin therapy

### 5.1 Personalized aspirin therapy

Pharmacogenetic testing has emerged as a promising approach to optimizing medical treatments by taking an individual's genetic makeup into account. This tailored approach involves analyzing a patient's genetic information to pinpoint specific genetic variations that might influence their response to medications, including aspirin. By gaining a deeper understanding of a person's genetic profile, healthcare professionals can finely adjust aspirin therapy to maximize its efficacy while minimizing potential adverse effects.

One of the key applications of pharmacogenetic testing in the context of aspirin therapy revolves around personalized dosing. Genetic variations in crucial drug-metabolizing enzymes, such as cytochrome P450 2C19 (CYP2C19), can substantially impact the way the body processes aspirin. Notably, patients harboring certain genetic variants might necessitate either higher or lower doses of aspirin to achieve the intended antiplatelet effect [179]. This adaptation in dosage takes into consideration an individual's genetic predisposition for metabolizing the drug, thereby aiming to optimize aspirin's impact on platelet aggregation.

Pharmacogenetic testing also offers a means of identifying individuals who might be predisposed to certain challenges during aspirin therapy. For instance, specific genetic variants within platelet receptors or polymorphisms within the COX-1 gene, responsible for cyclooxygenase-1 production, could lead to reduced responsiveness to aspirin or an elevated susceptibility to adverse reactions. By identifying these individuals through genetic testing, healthcare providers can proactively tailor treatment plans. This might involve considering alternative medications or modifying dosages to ensure an optimal response while minimizing risks [180, 181].

### 5.2 Reducing adverse events

Aspirin is generally regarded as a safe and well-tolerated medication, but it's important to recognize that certain individuals might encounter adverse events, such as gastrointestinal bleeding or hypersensitivity reactions. In this context, pharmacogenetic testing emerges as a valuable tool for identifying patients who could be at an elevated risk of experiencing such adverse events, thereby informing appropriate clinical decisions.

One notable application of pharmacogenetic testing is in identifying patients who might be more susceptible to aspirin-related gastrointestinal bleeding. Individuals harboring specific genetic variants within drug-metabolizing enzymes might have an increased predisposition to this adverse effect. By utilizing genetic profiling to identify these patients, healthcare providers gain the ability to implement preventive measures or explore alternative medication options to minimize the risk of gastrointestinal bleeding [182]. This tailored approach is particularly advantageous in ensuring patient safety while optimizing the therapeutic benefits of aspirin.

Moreover, genetic testing can play a crucial role in identifying individuals at a higher risk of hypersensitivity reactions to aspirin, such as those with aspirin-exacerbated respiratory disease (AERD). By recognizing these patients through genetic analysis, healthcare providers can avoid prescribing aspirin to them. This proactive measure helps prevent potentially severe allergic reactions and enables healthcare professionals to explore alternative treatment strategies that will not trigger adverse reactions [183].

### 5.3 Improving cardiovascular outcomes

Cardiovascular diseases (CVDs), including heart attacks and strokes, are significant health concerns on a global scale. Among the interventions for managing these conditions, aspirin emerges as a crucial player in the secondary prevention of CVDs. By reducing the risk of recurring cardiovascular events, aspirin has established its importance. However, it's important to recognize that aspirin's effectiveness might exhibit variability influenced by an individual's unique genetic composition.

Pharmacogenomic insights, obtained through genetic testing, offer a pathway to identifying individuals who are more likely to derive substantial benefits from aspirin therapy in the context of cardiovascular event prevention. Genetic testing provides healthcare professionals with valuable information that helps them recognize patients who could experience enhanced advantages from aspirin treatment. For instance, patients harboring specific genetic variants linked to heightened platelet aggregation or increased inflammation might experience more pronounced benefits from aspirin therapy. This knowledge empowers healthcare providers to offer a targeted approach to these patients, tailoring their treatment to optimize outcomes.

Conversely, genetic variations can also lead to reduced responsiveness to aspirin, a phenomenon known as aspirin resistance. Identifying individuals who possess these genetic variants is pivotal in guiding clinical decisions. Healthcare providers armed with this genetic information can consider alternative treatment strategies for patients who might not respond optimally to aspirin. This proactive approach ensures that patients receive the most suitable therapies to achieve the best possible health outcomes [184].

## 6. Conclusion

Aspirin, a widely used medication dating back to 1904, holds a prominent place in the medical world. Originally known for its pain-relieving, anti-inflammatory, and fever-reducing properties, its applications have expanded over the years, particularly in secondary prevention for cardiovascular disease. Additionally, its anti-inflammatory attributes have led to exploration in preventing inflammation-related cancers like colon cancer. With its low cost and extensive clinical experience, aspirin is now being investigated in various fields, including neurological diseases, virus-associated conditions, and bone physiology.

Despite its widespread use, the evaluation of aspirin's benefits and potential harms is essential, as it may lead to severe bleeding or damage to the stomach mucosa. To unlock its full potential, ongoing research on the molecular mechanisms of aspirin's action is uncovering predictive biomarkers. This newfound understanding allows for targeted, safer, and more effective use of this simple yet powerful medication.

In the realm of personalized medicine, the integration of pharmacogenetic and pharmacogenomic information into aspirin therapy represents a significant advancement. By tailoring aspirin treatment based on an individual's genetic profile, precise dosing can be achieved, resulting in improved treatment outcomes and better management of aspirin-related challenges. As personalized medicine continues to progress, its application holds great promise for shaping the future of aspirin therapy, benefitting patients in cardiovascular disease management and other areas.

To fully realize these advancements, collaborative efforts between researchers, clinicians, and policymakers are vital. By working together, these findings can be translated into routine clinical practice, ultimately optimizing aspirin's therapeutic benefits and enhancing patient care in a wide range of medical scenarios.

## Acknowledgements

The authors express their sincere thanks to the Faculty of Pharmacy, Integral University, Lucknow for encouraging and providing research atmosphere.

## Conflict of interest

The authors declare no conflict of interest.

## Author details

Mohd Aftab Siddiqui[1*], Charul Jain[1], Afreen Usmani[2], Abdul Hafeez[1], Mohammad Khalid[3] and Mohd Mujahid[4]

1 Department of Pharmacy, Integral University, Lucknow, U.P., India

2 Umapati Mahadev College of Pharmacy, Amroha, U.P., India

3 College of Pharmacy, Prince Sattam Bin Abdulaziz University Alkharj, Riyadh, Saudi Arabia

4 College of Pharmacy, University of Hafr Al-Batin, Saudi Arabia

*Address all correspondence to: aftab.uzaiz@gmail.com

## References

[1] Moyad MA. An introduction to aspirin, NSAIDs, and COX-2 inhibitors for the primary prevention of cardiovascular events and cancer and their potential preventive role in bladder carcinogenesis: Part I. InSeminars in Urologic Oncology. 2001;**19**(4):294-305

[2] Wood JN. From plant extract to molecular panacea: A commentary on stone (1763)'an account of the success of the bark of the willow in the cure of the agues'. Philosophical Transactions of the Royal Society B: Biological Sciences. 2015;**370**(1666):20140317

[3] Dreser H. Pharmakologisches über aspirin (acetylsalicylsäure). Archiv für die gesamte Physiologie des Menschen und der Tiere. 1899;**76**(5-6):306-318

[4] Salicylate (Oral Route, Rectal Route) [Internet]. Mayoclinic.org. 2023 [cited 2023 Jan 30]. Available from: https://www.mayoclinic.org/drugs-supplements/salicylate-oral-route-rectal-route/description/drg-20070551

[5] Patrono C, Baigent C. Role of aspirin in primary prevention of cardiovascular disease. Nature Reviews Cardiology. 2019;**16**(11):675-686

[6] Capodanno D, Angiolillo DJ. Aspirin for primary cardiovascular risk prevention and beyond in diabetes mellitus. Circulation. 2016;**134**(20):1579-1594

[7] Catella-Lawson F, Reilly MP, Kapoor SC, Cucchiara AJ, DeMarco S, Tournier B, et al. Cyclooxygenase inhibitors and the antiplatelet effects of aspirin. New England Journal of Medicine. 2001;**345**(25):1809-1817

[8] Olsen AM, Gislason GH, McGettigan P, Fosbøl E, Sørensen R, Hansen ML, et al. Association of NSAID use with risk of bleeding and cardiovascular events in patients receiving antithrombotic therapy after myocardial infarction. Journal of the American Medical Association. 2015;**313**(8):805-814

[9] Montinari MR, Minelli S, De Caterina R. The first 3500 years of aspirin history from its roots–a concise summary. Vascular pharmacology. 2019;**113**:1-8

[10] Gorelick PB, Born GV, D'Agostino RB, Hanley DF Jr, Moye L, Pepine CJ. Therapeutic benefit: Aspirin revisited in light of the introduction of clopidogrel. Stroke. 1999;**30**(8):1716-1721

[11] Garavito RM, Mulichak AM. The structure of mammalian cyclooxygenases. Annual review of biophysics and biomolecular structure. 2003;**32**(1):183-206

[12] Tóth L, Muszbek L, Komáromi I. Mechanism of the irreversible inhibition of human cyclooxygenase-1 by aspirin as predicted by QM/MM calculations. Journal of Molecular Graphics and Modelling. 2013;**40**:99-109

[13] Alfonso L, Ai G, Spitale RC, Bhat GJ. Molecular targets of aspirin and cancer prevention. British Journal of Cancer. 2014;111(1):61-67.

[14] Cipollone F, Patrignani P, Greco A, Panara MR, Padovano R, Cuccurullo F, et al. Differential suppression of thromboxane biosynthesis by indobufen and aspirin in patients with unstable angina. Circulation. 1997;**96**(4):1109-1116

[15] Patrono C. Aspirin: New cardiovascular uses for an old drug. The American journal of medicine. 2001;**110**(1):S62-S65

[16] Pradono P, Tazawa R, Maemondo M, Tanaka M, Usui K, Saijo Y, et al. Gene transfer of thromboxane A2 synthase and prostaglandin I2 synthase antithetically altered tumor angiogenesis and tumor growth. Cancer Research. 2002;**62**(1):63-66

[17] Baigent C, Blackwell L, Collins R, Emberson J, Godwin J, Peto R, et al. Aspirin in the primary and secondary prevention of vascular disease: Collaborative meta-analysis of individual participant data from randomised trials. Lancet. 2009;**373**(9678):1849-1860

[18] Mount M, Toltzis P. 50 years ago in the journal of Pediatrics: Aspirin and Reye syndrome. The Journal of Pediatrics. 2020;**222**:192

[19] Sindrup SH, Brøsen K, Gram LF. The relationship between sparteine oxidation polymorphism and steady-state kinetics of sparteine and its major metabolites. Clinical Pharmacology and Therapeutics. 1991;**50**(1):23-32

[20] Eikelboom JW, Hankey GJ, Thom J, Bhatt DL, Steg PG, Montalescot G, et al. Incomplete inhibition of thromboxane biosynthesis by acetylsalicylic acid: Determinants and effect on cardiovascular risk. Circulation. 2008;**118**(17):1705-1712

[21] Voora D, Cyr D, Lucas J, et al. Aspirin exposure reveals novel genes associated with platelet function and cardiovascular events. Journal of the American College of Cardiology. 2013;**62**(14):1267-1276

[22] Laidlaw TM, Cahill KN. Current knowledge and management of hypersensitivity to aspirin and NSAIDs. The Journal of Allergy and Clinical Immunology: In Practice. 2017;**5**(3):537-545

[23] Gollapudi RR, Teirstein PS, Stevenson DD, Simon RA. Aspirin sensitivity: Implications for patients with coronary artery disease. Journal of the American Medical Association. 2004;**292**(24):3017-3023

[24] Lee J. Aspirin desensitization as a treatment for aspirin-sensitive chronic spontaneous urticaria. Dermatologic Therapy. 2015;**28**(1):4-6

[25] Hankey GJ, Eikelboom JW. Aspirin resistance. The Lancet. 2006;**367**(9510):606-617

[26] Mansour K, Taher AT, Musallam KM, Alam S. Aspirin resistance. Advances in Hematology. 2009;**1**(1):1-10

[27] Volans GN. Effects of food and exercise on the absorption of effervescent aspirin. British Journal of Clinical Pharmacology. 1974;**1**(2):137

[28] Garabedian-Ruffalo SM, Syrja-Farber M, Lanius PM, Plucinski A. Monitoring of drug-drug and drug-food interactions. American Journal of Hospital Pharmacy. 1988;**45**(7):1530-1534

[29] Awwad S, Mohamed Ahmed AH, Sharma G, Heng JS, Khaw PT, Brocchini S, et al. Principles of pharmacology in the eye. British Journal of Pharmacology. 2017;**174**(23):4205-4223

[30] García Rodríguez LA, Martín-Pérez M, Hennekens CH, Rothwell PM, Lanas A. Bleeding risk with long-term low-dose aspirin: A systematic review of observational studies. PLoS One. 2016;**11**(8):e0160046

[31] Mohapatra TK, Subudhi BB. Repurposing of aspirin: Opportunities and challenges. Research Journal of Pharmacy and Technology. 2019;**12**(4):2037-2044

[32] Gartner AH. Aspirin-induced gastritis and gastrointestinal bleeding. The Journal of the American Dental Association. 1976;**93**(1):111-117

[33] Chapman J, Arnold JK. Reye syndrome. In: StatPearls. Treasure Island, FL: StatPearls Publishing; 2018

[34] Uppala R, Dudiak B, Beck ME, Bharathi SS, Zhang Y, Stolz DB, et al. Aspirin increases mitochondrial fatty acid oxidation. Biochemical and Biophysical Research Communications. 2017;**482**(2):346-351

[35] Schrör K. Aspirin and Reye syndrome: A review of the evidence. Pediatric Drugs. 2007;**9**:195-204

[36] Doutremepuich C, Aguejouf O, Desplat V, Eizayaga FX. Aspirin discontinuation syndromes: Clinical implications of basic research studies. American Journal of Cardiovascular Drugs. 2013;**13**:377-384

[37] Ferrari E, Benhamou M, Cerboni P, Marcel B. Coronary syndromes following aspirin withdrawal: A special risk for late stent thrombosis. Journal of the American College of Cardiology. 2005;**45**(3):456-459

[38] Sundström J, Hedberg J, Thuresson M, Aarskog P, Johannesen KM, Oldgren J. Low-dose aspirin discontinuation and risk of cardiovascular events: A Swedish nationwide, population-based cohort study. Circulation. 2017;**136**(13):1183-1192

[39] Davies MJ, Thomas AC. Plaque fissuring--the cause of acute myocardial infarction, sudden ischaemic death, and crescendo angina. British Heart Journal. 1985;**53**(4):363

[40] Gaglia MA Jr, Clavijo L. Cardiovascular pharmacology core reviews: Aspirin. Journal of Cardiovascular Pharmacology and Therapeutics. 2013;**18**(6):505-513

[41] Members TF, Montalescot G, Sechtem U, Achenbach S, Andreotti F, Arden C, et al. 2013 ESC guidelines on the management of stable coronary artery disease: The task force on the management of stable coronary artery disease of the European Society of Cardiology. European Heart Journal. 2013;**34**(38):2949-3003

[42] Paikin JS, Eikelboom JW. Aspirin. Circulation. 2012;**125**(10):e439-e442

[43] ISIS-2 Collaborative Group. Randomized trial of intravenous streptokinase, oral aspirin, both, or neither among 17,187 cases of suspected acute myocardial infarction. ISIS-2. Lancet. 1988;**1**:49-360

[44] del Zoppo GJ, Hallenbeck JM. Advances in the vascular pathophysiology of ischemic stroke. Thrombosis Research. 2000;**98**(3):73-81

[45] Goertler M, Baeumer M, Kross R, Blaser T, Lutze G, Jost S, et al. Rapid decline of cerebral microemboli of arterial origin after intravenous acetylsalicylic acid. Stroke. 1999;**30**(1):66-69

[46] Dyken ML, Barnett HJ, Easton JD, Fields WS, Fuster V, Hachinski V, et al. Low-dose aspirin and stroke." it ain't necessarily so". Stroke. 1992;**23**(10):1395-1399

[47] Dutch TIA Trial Study Group*. A comparison of two doses of aspirin (30

mg vs. 283 mg a day) in patients after a transient ischemic attack or minor ischemic stroke. New England Journal of Medicine. 1991;**325**(18):1261-1266

[48] Uk-Tia Study Group. United Kingdom transient ischaemic attack (UK-TIA) aspirin trial: Interim results. British Medical Journal (Clinical Research Ed.). 1988;**296**(6618):316-320

[49] Jauch EC, Saver JL, Adams HP Jr, Bruno A, Connors JJ, Demaerschalk BM, et al. Guidelines for the early management of patients with acute ischemic stroke: A guideline for healthcare professionals from the American Heart Association/ American Stroke Association. Stroke. 2013;**44**(3):870-947

[50] Maulaz AB, Bezerra DC, Michel P, Bogousslavsky J. Effect of discontinuing aspirin therapy on the risk of brain ischemic stroke. Archives of Neurology. 2005;**62**(8):1217-1220

[51] Bachman DS. Discontinuing chronic aspirin therapy: Another risk factor for stroke? Annals of Neurology: Official Journal of the American Neurological Association and the Child Neurology Society. 2002;**51**(1):137-138

[52] Sibon I, Orgogozo JM. Antiplatelet drug discontinuation is a risk factor for ischemic stroke. Neurology. 2004;**62**(7):1187-1189

[53] Burger W, Chemnitius JM, Kneissl GD, Rücker G. Low-dose aspirin for secondary cardiovascular prevention–cardiovascular risks after its perioperative withdrawal versus bleeding risks with its continuation–review and meta-analysis. Journal of Internal Medicine. 2005;**257**(5):399-414

[54] Weitz JI, Byrne J, Clagett GP, Farkouh ME, Porter JM, Sackett DL, et al. Diagnosis and treatment of chronic arterial insufficiency of the lower extremities: A critical review. Circulation. 1996;**94**(11):3026-3049

[55] Hiatt WR. Preventing atherothrombotic events in peripheral arterial disease: The use of antiplatelet therapy. Journal of Internal Medicine. 2002;**251**(3):193-206

[56] Matsagas MI, Geroulakos G, Mikhailidis DP. The role of platelets in peripheral arterial disease: Therapeutic implications. Annals of Vascular Surgery. 2002;**16**(2):246-258

[57] Koksch M, Zeiger F, Wittig K, Siegemund A, Reininger CB, Pfeiffer D, et al. Coagulation, fibrinolysis and platelet P-selectin expression in peripheral vascular disease. European Journal of Vascular and Endovascular Surgery. 2001;**21**(2):147-154

[58] Tsakiris DA, Tschöpl M, Jäger K, Haefeli WE, Wolf F, Marbet GA. Circulating cell adhesion molecules and endothelial markers before and after transluminal angioplasty in peripheral arterial occlusive disease. Atherosclerosis. 1999;**142**(1):193-200

[59] Zahavi J, Zahavi M. Enhanced platelet release reaction, shortened platelet survival time and increased platelet aggregation and plasma thromboxane B2 in chronic obstructive arterial disease. Thrombosis and Haemostasis. 1985;**53**(01):105-109

[60] Reininger CB, Boeger CA, Steckmeier B, Spannagl M, Schweiberer L. Mechanisms underlying increased platelet reactivity in patients with peripheral arterial disease: Preliminary results. International Angiology. 1999;**18**(2):163

[61] Reininger CB, Graf J, Reininger AJ, Spannagl M, Steckmeier B, Schweiberer L.

Increased platelet and coagulatory activity in peripheral atherosclerosis flow mediated platelet function is a sensitive and specific disease indicator. International Angiology: a Journal of the International Union of Angiology. 1996;**15**(4):335-343

[62] Schrör K, Zimmermann KC, Tannhäuser R. Augmented myocardial ischaemia by nicotine–mechanisms and their possible significance. British Journal of Pharmacology. 1998;**125**(1):79

[63] Roller RE, Dorr A, Ulrich S, Pilger E. Effect of aspirin treatment in patients with peripheral arterial disease monitored with the platelet function analyzer PFA-100. Blood Coagulation & Fibrinolysis. 2002;**13**(4):277-281

[64] Mueller MR, Salat A, Stangl P, Murabito M, Pulaki S, Boehm D, et al. Variable platelet response to low-dose ASA and the risk of limb deterioration in patients submitted to peripheral arterial angioplasty. Thrombosis and Haemostasis. 1997;**78**(09):1003-1007

[65] Walters TK, Mitchell DC, Wood RF. Low-dose aspirin fails to inhibit increased platelet reactivity in patients with peripheral vascular disease. Journal of British Surgery. 1993;**80**(10):1266-1268

[66] Van Geffen JP, Kleinegris MC, Verdoold R, Baaten CC, Cosemans JM, Clemetson KJ, et al. Normal platelet activation profile in patients with peripheral arterial disease on aspirin. Thrombosis Research. 2015;**135**(3):513-520

[67] Armstrong EJ, Chen DC, Westin GG, Singh S, McCoach CE, Bang H, et al. Adherence to guideline-recommended therapy is associated with decreased major adverse cardiovascular events and major adverse limb events among patients with peripheral arterial disease. Journal of the American Heart Association. 2014;**3**(2):e000697

[68] Rosendaal FR. Venous thrombosis: A multicausal disease. The Lancet. 1999;**353**(9159):1167-1173

[69] Wallén NH, Ladjevardi M. Influence of low-and high-dose aspirin treatment on thrombin generation in whole blood. Thrombosis Research. 1998;**92**(4):189-194

[70] Szczeklik A, Krzanowski M, Gora P, Radwan J. Antiplatelet drugs and generation of thrombin in clotting blood. 1992. pp. 2006-2011

[71] Undas A, Undas R, Musiał J, Szczeklik A. A low dose of aspirin (75 mg/day) lowers thrombin generation to a similar extent as a high dose of aspirin (300 mg/day). Blood Coagulation & Fibrinolysis: an International Journal in Haemostasis and Thrombosis. 2000;**11**(3):231-234

[72] Becattini C, Agnelli G, Schenone A, Eichinger S, Bucherini E, Silingardi M, et al. Aspirin for preventing the recurrence of venous thromboembolism. New England Journal of Medicine. 2012;**366**(21):1959-1967

[73] Brighton TA, Eikelboom JW, Mann K, Mister R, Gallus A, Ockelford P, et al. Low-dose aspirin for preventing recurrent venous thromboembolism. The New England Journal of Medicine. 2012;**367**:1979-1987

[74] Hashemi V, Dolati S, Hosseini A, Gharibi T, Danaii S, Yousefi M. Natural killer T cells in preeclampsia: An updated review. Biomedicine & Pharmacotherapy. 2017;**95**:412-418

[75] Eghbal-Fard S, Yousefi M, Heydarlou H, Ahmadi M, Taghavi S,

Movasaghpour A, et al. The imbalance of Th17/Treg axis involved in the pathogenesis of preeclampsia. Journal of Cellular Physiology. 2019;**234**(4):5106-5116

[76] Klockenbusch W, Goecke TW, Krüssel JS, Tutschek BA, Crombach G, Schrör K. Prostacyclin deficiency and reduced fetoplacental blood flow in pregnancy-induced hypertension and preeclampsia. Gynecologic and Obstetric Investigation. 2000;**50**(2):103-107

[77] Briel RC, Kieback DG, Lippert TH. Platelet sensitivity to a prostacyclin analogue in normal and pathological pregnancy. Prostaglandins, Leukotrienes and Medicine. 1984;**13**(3):335-340

[78] Klockenbusch W, Hohlfeld T, Wilhelm M, Somville T, Schrör K. Platelet PGI2 receptor affinity is reduced in pre-eclampsia. British journal of Clinical Pharmacology. 1996;**41**(6):616-618

[79] Redman CW, Bonnar J, Beilin LJ. Early platelet consumption in pre-eclampsia. British Medical Journal. 1978;**1**(6111):467-469

[80] Van Assche FA, Spitz B, Vermylen J, Deckmijn H. Preliminary observations on treatment of pregnancy-induced hypertension with a thromboxane synthetase inhibitor. American Journal of Obstetrics and Gynecology. 1984;**148**(2):216-218

[81] Sullivan MH, Clark NA, De Swiet M, Nelson-Piercy C, Elder MG. Titration of antiplatelet treatment in pregnant women at risk of preeclampsia. Thrombosis and Haemostasis. 1998;**79**(04):743-746

[82] Carbillon L, Uzan S. Early treatment with low-dose aspirin is effective for the prevention of preeclampsia and related complications in high-risk patients selected by the analysis of their historic risk factors. Blood. 2005;**105**(2):902-903

[83] Park F, Russo K, Pellosi M, Puddephat R, Walter M, Leung R, et al. The impact of aspirin on the prevalence of early onset pre-eclampsia after first trimester screening. Prenatal Diagnosis. 2014;**34**(Suppl 1):e4

[84] Duley L, Henderson-Smart D, Knight M, King J. Antiplatelet drugs for prevention of pre-eclampsia and its consequences: Systematic review. BMJ. 2001;**322**(7282):329-333

[85] Porter TF, Gyamfi-Bannerman C, Manuck T. Low-dose aspirin use during pregnancy. Obstetrics and Gynecology. 2018;**132**(1):E44-E52

[86] Askie LM, Duley L, Henderson-Smart DJ, Stewart LA. Antiplatelet agents for prevention of pre-eclampsia: A meta-analysis of individual patient data. The Lancet. 2007;**369**(9575):1791-1798

[87] El-Achi V, Park F, O'Brien C, Tooher J, Hyett J. Does low dose aspirin prescribed for risk of early onset preeclampsia reduce the prevalence of preterm prelabor rupture of membranes? The Journal of Maternal-Fetal & Neonatal Medicine. 2021;**34**(4):618-623

[88] Heyborne KD. Preeclampsia prevention: Lessons from the low-dose aspirin therapy trials. American Journal of Obstetrics and Gynecology. 2000;**183**(3):523-528

[89] Merviel P, Carbillon L, Challier JC, Rabreau M, Beaufils M, Uzan S. Pathophysiology of preeclampsia: Links with implantation disorders. European Journal of Obstetrics & Gynecology and Reproductive Biology. 2004;**115**(2):134-147

[90] Ye X, Fu J, Yang Y, Gao Y, Liu L, Chen S. Frequency-risk and duration-risk relationships between aspirin use and gastric cancer: A systematic

review and meta-analysis. PLoS One. 2013;**8**(7):e71522

[91] Colussi D, Brandi G, Bazzoli F, Ricciardiello L. Molecular pathways involved in colorectal cancer: Implications for disease behavior and prevention. International Journal of Molecular Sciences. 2013;**14**(8):16365-16385

[92] Liang J, Nagahashi M, Kim EY, Harikumar KB, Yamada A, Huang WC, et al. Sphingosine-1-phosphate links persistent STAT3 activation, chronic intestinal inflammation, and development of colitis-associated cancer. Cancer Cell. 2013;**23**(1):107-120

[93] Ponnusamy S, Meyers-Needham M, Senkal CE, Saddoughi SA, Sentelle D, Selvam SP, et al. Sphingolipids and cancer: Ceramide and sphingosine-1-phosphate in the regulation of cell death and drug resistance. Future Oncology. 2010;**6**(10):1603-1624

[94] Pyne NJ, Pyne S. Sphingosine 1-phosphate and cancer. Nature Reviews Cancer. 2010;**10**(7):489-503

[95] Cook NR, Lee IM, Zhang SM, Moorthy MV, Buring JE. Alternate-day, low-dose aspirin and cancer risk: Long-term observational follow-up of a randomized trial. Annals of Internal Medicine. 2013;**159**(2):77-85

[96] Patrono C, Ciabattoni G, Pinca E, Pugliese F, Castrucci G, De Salvo A, et al. Low dose aspirin and inhibition of thromboxane B2 production in healthy subjects. Thrombosis Research. 1980;**17**(3-4):317-327

[97] Chan TA, Morin PJ, Vogelstein B, Kinzler KW. Mechanisms underlying nonsteroidal antiinflammatory drug-mediated apoptosis. National Academy of Sciences of the United States of America. 1998;**95**(2):681-686

[98] Chan AT, Giovannucci EL, Meyerhardt JA, Schernhammer ES, Curhan GC, Fuchs CS. Long-term use of aspirin and nonsteroidal anti-inflammatory drugs and risk of colorectal cancer. Journal of the American Medical Association. 2005;**294**(8):914-923

[99] Egan KM, Stampfer MJ, Giovannucci E, Rosner BA, Colditz GA. Prospective study of regular aspirin use and the risk of breast cancer. JNCI: Journal of the National Cancer Institute. 1996;**88**(14):988-993

[100] Mann B, Gelos M, Siedow A, Hanski ML, Gratchev A, Ilyas M, et al. Target genes of β-catenin–T cell-factor/lymphoid-enhancer-factor signaling in human colorectal carcinomas. National Academy of Sciences of the United States of America. 1999;**96**(4):1603-1608

[101] Bos CL, Kodach LL, van den Brink GR, Diks SH, van Santen MM, Richel DJ, et al. Effect of aspirin on the Wnt/β-catenin pathway is mediated via protein phosphatase 2A. Oncogene. 2006;**25**(49):6447-6456

[102] Chen Z, Hagler J, Palombella VJ, Melandri F, Scherer D, Ballard D, et al. Signal-induced site-specific phosphorylation targets I kappa B alpha to the ubiquitin-proteasome pathway. Genes & Development. 1995;**9**(13):1586-1597

[103] Yin MJ, Yamamoto Y, Gaynor RB. The anti-inflammatory agents aspirin and salicylate inhibit the activity of IκB kinase-β. Nature. 1998;**396**(6706):77-80

[104] Kune GA, Kune S, Watson LF. Colorectal cancer risk, chronic illnesses, operations, and medications: Case control results from the Melbourne colorectal cancer study. Cancer Research. 1988;**48**(15):4399-4404

[105] Bosetti C, Rosato V, Gallus S, Cuzick J, La Vecchia C. Aspirin and cancer risk: A quantitative review to 2011. Annals of Oncology. 2012;**23**(6):1403-1415

[106] Bibbins-Domingo K. US preventive services task force. Aspirin use for the primary prevention of cardiovascular disease and colorectal cancer: US preventive services task force recommendation statement. Annals of Internal Medicine. 2016;**164**(12):836-845

[107] Fraser DM, Sullivan FM, Thompson AM, McCowan C. Aspirin use and survival after the diagnosis of breast cancer: A population-based cohort study. British Journal of Cancer. 2014;**111**(3):623-627

[108] Cossack M, Ghaffary C, Watson P, Snyder C, Lynch H. Aspirin use is associated with lower prostate cancer risk in male carriers of BRCA mutations. Journal of Genetic Counseling. 2014;**23**(2):187-191

[109] Downer MK, Allard CB, Preston MA, Gaziano JM, Stampfer MJ, Mucci LA, et al. Regular aspirin use and the risk of lethal prostate cancer in the physicians' health study. European Urology. 2017;**72**(5):821-827

[110] Brotons C, Benamouzig R, Filipiak KJ, Limmroth V, Borghi C. A systematic review of aspirin in primary prevention: Is it time for a new approach? American Journal of Cardiovascular Drugs. 2015;**15**:113-133

[111] Querfurth HW, LaFerla FM. Alzheimer's disease. New England Journal of Medicine. 2010;**362**(4):329-344

[112] Mattson MP. Pathways towards and away from Alzheimer's disease. Nature. 2004;**430**(7000):631-639

[113] Schrör K. Acetylsalicylic Acid. Hoboken, New Jersey: John Wiley & Sons; 2016

[114] Jiang Q, Lee CD, Mandrekar S, Wilkinson B, Cramer P, Zelcer N, et al. ApoE promotes the proteolytic degradation of Aβ. Neuron. 2008;**58**(5):681-693

[115] Koistinaho M, Koistinaho J. Interactions between Alzheimer's disease and cerebral ischemia—Focus on inflammation. Brain Research Reviews. 2005;**48**(2):240-250

[116] Chen M, Inestrosa NC, Ross GS, Fernandez HL. Platelets are the primary source of amyloid β-peptide in human blood. Biochemical and Biophysical Research Communications. 1995;**213**(1):96-103

[117] Tang K, Hynan LS, Baskin F, Rosenberg RN. Platelet amyloid precursor protein processing: A bio-marker for Alzheimer's disease. Journal of the Neurological Sciences. 2006;**240**(1-2):53-58

[118] Lue LF, Kuo YM, Roher AE, Brachova L, Shen Y, Sue L, et al. Soluble amyloid β peptide concentration as a predictor of synaptic change in Alzheimer's disease. The American Journal of Pathology. 1999;**155**(3):853-862

[119] Medeiros R, Kitazawa M, Passos GF, Baglietto-Vargas D, Cheng D, Cribbs DH, et al. Aspirin-triggered lipoxin A4 stimulates alternative activation of microglia and reduces Alzheimer disease–like pathology in mice. The American Journal of Pathology. 2013;**182**(5):1780-1789

[120] Harris JR. In vitro fibrillogenesis of the amyloid β1-42 peptide: Cholesterol potentiation and aspirin inhibition. Micron. 2002;**33**(7-8):609-626

[121] Hirohata M, Ono K, Naiki H, Yamada M. Non-steroidal anti-inflammatory drugs have anti-amyloidogenic effects for Alzheimer's β-amyloid fibrils in vitro. Neuropharmacology. 2005;**49**(7):1088-1099

[122] Alexopoulos GS, Jeste DV, Chung H, Carpenter D, Ross R, Docherty JP. The expert consensus guideline series. Treatment of dementia and its behavioral disturbances. Introduction: Methods, commentary, and summary. Postgraduate Medicine. Jan 2005. Spec No. 6-22

[123] Iqbal K, Grundke-Iqbal I. Developing pharmacological therapies for Alzheimer disease. Cellular and Molecular Life Sciences. 2007;**64**:2234-2244

[124] Berk M, Dean O, Drexhage H, McNeil JJ, Moylan S, O'Neil A, et al. Aspirin: A review of its neurobiological properties and therapeutic potential for mental illness. BMC Medicine. 2013;**11**(1):1-7

[125] Hybiak J, Broniarek I, Kiryczyński G, Los LD, Rosik J, Machaj F, et al. Aspirin and its pleiotropic application. European Journal of Pharmacology. 2020;**866**:172762

[126] Klok FA, Kruip MJ, Van der Meer NJ, Arbous MS, Gommers DA, Kant KM, et al. Incidence of thrombotic complications in critically ill ICU patients with COVID-19. Thrombosis Research. 2020;**191**:145-147

[127] Elbadawi A, Elgendy IY, Sahai A, Bhandari R, McCarthy M, Gomes M, et al. Incidence and outcomes of thrombotic events in symptomatic patients with COVID-19. Arteriosclerosis, Thrombosis, and Vascular Biology. 2021;**41**(1):545-547

[128] Bekelis K, Missios S, Ahmad J, Labropoulos N, Schirmer CM, Calnan DR, et al. Ischemic stroke occurs less frequently in patients with COVID-19: A multicenter cross-sectional study. Stroke. 2020;**51**(12):3570-3576

[129] Ellul MA, Benjamin L, Singh B, Lant S, Michael BD, Easton A, et al. Neurological associations of COVID-19. The Lancet Neurology. 2020;**19**(9):767-783

[130] Di Minno A, Ambrosino P, Calcaterra I, Di Minno MN. COVID-19 and venous thromboembolism: A meta-analysis of literature studies. In: Seminars in Thrombosis and Hemostasis. Vol. 46, No. 07. New York, NY, USA: Thieme Medical Publishers; 3 Sep 2020. pp. 763-771

[131] McBane II RD, Roldan VD, Niven AS, Pruthi RK, Franco PM, Linderbaum JA, et al. Anticoagulation in COVID-19: A systematic review, meta-analysis, and rapid guidance from Mayo Clinic. In: Mayo Clinic Proceedings. Vol. 95, No. 11. Amsterdam: Elsevier; 1 Nov 2020. pp. 2467-2486

[132] Tang N, Bai H, Chen X, Gong J, Li D, Sun Z. Anticoagulant treatment is associated with decreased mortality in severe coronavirus disease 2019 patients with coagulopathy. Journal of thrombosis and haemostasis. 2020;**18**(5):1094-1099

[133] Manne BK, Denorme F, Middleton EA, Portier I, Rowley JW, Stubben C, et al. Platelet gene expression and function in patients with COVID-19. Blood. 2020;**136**(11):1317-1329

[134] Zaid Y, Puhm F, Allaeys I, Naya A, Oudghiri M, Khalki L, et al. Platelets can associate with SARS-Cov-2 RNA and are hyperactivated in COVID-19. Circulation research. 2020;**127**(11):1404-1418

[135] Hottz ED, Azevedo-Quintanilha IG, Palhinha L, Teixeira L, Barreto EA, Pão CR, et al. Platelet activation and platelet-monocyte aggregate formation trigger tissue factor expression in patients with severe COVID-19. Blood. 2020;**136**(11):1330-1341

[136] Barrett TJ, Lee A, Xia Y, Lin LH, Black M, Cotzia P, et al. Biomarkers of platelet activity and vascular health associate with thrombosis and mortality in patients with COVID-19. Circulation Research. 2020;**127**:945-947

[137] Wichmann D, Sperhake JP, Lütgehetmann M, et al. Autopsy findings and venous thromboembolism in patients with COVID-19: A prospective cohort study. Annals of Internal Medicine. 2020;**2020**(10):M20-M2003

[138] Glatthaar-Saalmüller B, Mair KH, Saalmüller A. Antiviral activity of aspirin against RNA viruses of the respiratory tract—An in vitro study. Influenza and Other Respiratory Viruses. 2017;**11**(1):85-92

[139] Nakatsugi S, Sugimoto N, Furukawa M. Effects of non-steroidal anti-inflammatory drugs on prostaglandin E2 production by cyclooxygenase-2 from endogenous and exogenous arachidonic acid in rat peritoneal macrophages stimulated with lipopolysaccharide. Prostaglandins, Leukotrienes and Essential Fatty Acids. 1996;**55**(6):451-457

[140] Wijaya I, Andhika R, Huang I, Purwiga A, Budiman KY. The effects of aspirin on the outcome of COVID-19: A systematic review and meta-analysis. Clinical Epidemiology and Global Health. 2021;**12**:100883

[141] Caspi D, Lubart E, Graff E, Habot B, Yaron M, Segal R. The effect of mini-dose aspirin on renal function and uric acid handling in elderly patients. Arthritis & Rheumatism: Official Journal of the American College of Rheumatology. 2000;**43**(1):103-108

[142] Segal R, Lubart E, Leibovitz A, Berkovitch M, Habot B, Yaron M, et al. Early and late effects of low-dose aspirin on renal function in elderly patients. The American Journal of Medicine. 2003;**115**(6):462-466

[143] D'Agati V. Does aspirin cause acute or chronic renal failure in experimental animals and in humans? American Journal of Kidney Diseases. 1996;**28**(1):S24-S29

[144] Thomas VP, Paul KW, Michael JK. Risk of kidney failure associated with the use of acetaminophen, aspirin, and nonsteroidal Antiinflammatory drugs. New England Journal of Medicine. 1994;**331**(25):1675-1679

[145] Winchester JF. Therapeutic uses of aspirin in renal diseases. American Journal of Kidney Diseases. 1996;**28**(1):S20-S23

[146] Zafarmand SS, Karimi-Haghighi S, Salehi MS, Hooshmandi E, Owjfard M, Bayat M, et al. Aspirin impacts on stem cells: Implications for therapeutic targets. Tissue and Cell. 2022;**74**:101707

[147] Deng L, Hu S, Baydoun AR, Chen J, Chen X, Cong X. Aspirin induces apoptosis in mesenchymal stem cells requiring Wnt/β-catenin pathway. Cell Proliferation. 2009;**42**(6):721-730

[148] Cao Y, Xiong J, Mei S, Wang F, Zhao Z, Wang S, et al. Aspirin promotes bone marrow mesenchymal stem cell-based calvarial bone regeneration in mini swine. Stem Cell Research & Therapy. 2015;**6**(1):1-1

[149] Yuan M, Zhan Y, Hu W, Li Y, Xie X, Miao N, et al. Aspirin promotes

osteogenic differentiation of human dental pulp stem cells. International Journal of Molecular Medicine. 2018;**42**(4):1967-1976

[150] Li Y, Luo Z, Xu X, Li Y, Zhang S, Zhou P, et al. Aspirin enhances the osteogenic and anti-inflammatory effects of human mesenchymal stem cells on osteogenic BFP-1 peptide-decorated substrates. Journal of Materials Chemistry B. 2017;**5**(34):7153-7163

[151] Newburger JW, Burns JC. Kawasaki disease. Vascular Medicine. 1999;**4**(3):187-202

[152] Baumer JH, Love S, Gupta A, Haines L, Maconochie IK, Dua JS. Salicylate for the treatment of Kawasaki disease in children. Cochrane Database of Systematic Reviews. 2006;**4**(1):1-5

[153] Kuo HC, Guo MM, Lo MH, Hsieh KS, Huang YH. Effectiveness of intravenous immunoglobulin alone and intravenous immunoglobulin combined with high-dose aspirin in the acute stage of Kawasaki disease: Study protocol for a randomized controlled trial. BMC Pediatrics. 2018;**18**(1):1-6

[154] Galeotti C, Bayry J, Kone-Paut I, Kaveri SV. Kawasaki disease: Aetiopathogenesis and therapeutic utility of intravenous immunoglobulin. Autoimmunity Reviews. 2010;**9**(6):441-448

[155] Newburger JW, Fulton DR. Kawasaki disease. Current Treatment Options in Cardiovascular Medicine. 2007;**9**(2):148-158

[156] Cambria-Kiely JA, Gandhi PJ. Aspirin resistance and genetic polymorphisms. Journal of Thrombosis and Thrombolysis. 2002;**14**:51-58

[157] Mega JL, Close SL, Wiviott SD, Shen L, Hockett RD, Brandt JT, et al. Cytochrome p-450 polymorphisms and response to clopidogrel. New England Journal of Medicine. 2009;**360**(4):354-362

[158] Wurtz M, Dalby Kristensen S, HvasAM,LerkevangGE.Pharmacogenetics of the antiplatelet effect of aspirin. Current Pharmaceutical Design. 2012;**18**(33):5294-5308

[159] Niemi M. Transporter pharmacogenetics and statin toxicity. Clinical Pharmacology & Therapeutics. 2017;**101**(3):391-394

[160] Pasanen MK, Backman JT, Neuvonen PJ, Niemi M. SLCO1B1 polymorphism markedly affects the pharmacokinetics of simvastatin acid. Pharmacogenetics and Genomics. 2006;**16**(12):873-879

[161] Tachibana-Iimori R, Tabara Y. Impact of SLCO1B1 genetic variation on the pharmacokinetics of statins. Journal of Pharmaceutical Health Care and Sciences. 2018;**4**(1):1-9

[162] Consortium IH, Altshuler DM, Gibbs RA, Peltonen L, Dermitzakis E. Integrating common and rare genetic variation in diverse human populations. Nature. 2010;**467**(7311):52-58

[163] Ho RH, Kim RB. Transporters and drug therapy: Implications for drug disposition and disease. Clinical Pharmacology & Therapeutics. 2005;**78**(3):260-277

[164] Cattaneo M, Lombardi R, Lecchi A, et al. P-glycoprotein and drug interactions in primary care. Internal and Emergency Medicine. 2007;**2**(3):239-247

[165] Ma Q, Lu AY. Pharmacogenetics, pharmacogenomics, and individualized medicine. Pharmacological Reviews. 2011;**63**(2):437-459

[166] Hauser IA, Kruck S, Gauer S, et al. ABCB1 genotype of the donor but not of the recipient is a major risk factor for cyclosporine-related nephrotoxicity after renal transplantation. Journal of the American Society of Nephrology. 2002;**13**(4):1073-1081

[167] Kim KA, Joo HJ, Lee HM, Park JY. Effect of ABCB1 (MDR1) haplotypes derived from G2677T/C3435T on the pharmacokinetics of amlodipine in healthy subjects. British Journal of Clinical Pharmacology. 2006;**61**(5):545-554

[168] Massberg S, Schulz C, Gawaz M. Role of platelets in the pathophysiology of acute coronary syndrome. Seminars in Vascular Medicine. 2003;**3**(2):147-162

[169] Nieswandt B, Watson SP. Platelet-collagen interaction: Is GPVI the central receptor? Blood. 2003;**102**(2):449-461

[170] Gresele P, Kleiman NS, Lopez JA, Page CP, editors. Platelets in Thrombotic and Non-Thrombotic Disorders: Pathophysiology, Pharmacology and Therapeutics: An Update. New York, NY, United States: Springer; 8 Mar 2017

[171] Undas A, Brummel-Ziedins KE, Mann KG. Antithrombotic properties of aspirin and resistance to aspirin: Beyond strictly antiplatelet actions. Blood. 2007;**109**(6):2285-2292

[172] Mänttäri M, Manninen V, Huttunen JK, et al. Platelet receptor function and response to low-dose aspirin in essential hypertension. Circulation. 1993;**88**(3):832-837

[173] Rothwell PM, Cook NR, Gaziano JM, et al. Effects of aspirin on risks of vascular events and cancer according to bodyweight and dose: Analysis of individual patient data from randomised trials. The Lancet. 2019;**393**(10170):2841-2853

[174] Takahashi H, Kashima T, Nomizo Y, et al. Influence of CYP2C9 genetic polymorphisms on the inhibition of platelet aggregation after treatment with a low maintenance dose of aspirin. Drug Metabolism and Pharmacokinetics. 2008;**23**(3):194-200

[175] Pancrudo J, Ouwehand WH, Ozaki R, et al. Platelet function analyzer (PFA)-100 closure time in bleeding disorders is influenced by both the high shear–dependent and the low shear–dependent adhesive functions of von Willebrand factor. British Journal of Haematology. 2008;**141**(5):596-605

[176] Al-Azzam SI, Alzoubi KH, Khabour OF, Tawalbeh D, Al-Azzeh O. The contribution of platelet glycoproteins (GPIa C807T and GPIba C-5T) and cyclooxygenase 2 (COX-2G-765C) polymorphisms to platelet response in patients treated with aspirin. Gene. 2013;**526**(2):118-121

[177] Undas A, Sanak M, Musial J, Szczeklik A. Platelet glycoprotein IIIa polymorphism, aspirin, and thrombin generation. The Lancet. 1999;**353**(9157):982-983

[178] Abderrazek F, Chakroun T, Addad F, Dridi Z, Gerotziafas G, Gamra H, et al. The GPIIIa PlA polymorphism and the platelet hyperactivity in Tunisian patients with stable coronary artery disease treated with aspirin. Thrombosis Research. 2010;**125**(6):e265-e268

[179] Brown SA, Pereira N. Pharmacogenomic impact of CYP2C19 variation on clopidogrel therapy in precision cardiovascular medicine. Journal of Personalized Medicine. 2018;**8**(1):8

[180] Yang Y, Lewis JP, Hulot JS, Scott SA. The pharmacogenetic control of antiplatelet response: Candidate genes and CYP2C19. Expert Opinion on Drug Metabolism & Toxicology. 2015;**11**(10):1599-1617

[181] Bonney PA, Yim B, Brinjikji W, Walcott BP. Pharmacogenomic considerations for antiplatelet agents: The era of precision medicine in stroke prevention and neurointerventional practice. Molecular Case Studies. 2019;**5**(2):a003731

[182] Lee RU, Stevenson DD. Aspirin-exacerbated respiratory disease: Evaluation and management. Allergy, Asthma & Immunology Research. 2011;**3**(1):3-10

[183] Baigent C, Holmes MV. Variability in aspirin efficacy: All in the genes? European Heart Journal. 2019;**40**(41):3393-3396

[184] Mason PJ, Jacobs AK, Freedman JE. Aspirin resistance and atherothrombotic disease. Journal of the American College of Cardiology. 2005;**46**(6):986-993

Chapter 3

# Advancements in Gene Therapy for Type 2 Diabetes: Insights from CRISPR Cas9 Mediated Gene Editing and Insulin Production

*Sairam Venkatraman, Srinivasan S. Tharun, Ashok Pavithra and Reddy Amala*


## Abstract

This literature presents a comprehensive overview of the application of CRISPR-based gene editing technology in the treatment of diabetes mellitus (DM). The introduction highlights the significance of DM as one of the oldest human diseases and the need for effective control to prevent potential consequences. It emphasizes the limitations of conventional medications for hyperglycemia and the challenges in achieving optimal glucose concentrations and minimizing long-term consequences. The abstract then delves into the advancements in CRISPR technology, discussing various delivery methods for the CRISPR-Cas complex, including non-viral vectors, viral vectors, and nanocarriers. The use of CRISPR-Cpf1 as an alternative to Cas9 is explored, highlighting its advantages and functionality. The abstract further explores the potential of CRISPR gene therapy and nanocarriers in treating DM, particularly targeting the NLRP3 inflammasome and downregulating the DPP-4 enzyme. Liposomal particles and lecithin nano-liposomal particles are discussed as efficient delivery systems for CRISPR/Cas9, with potential applications in T2DM treatment. The role of islet amyloid polypeptide (IAPP) in T2DM and its study using CRISPR Cas9-based gene editing technology is also presented. Overall, this abstract provides a comprehensive overview of the current advancements and potential applications of CRISPR technology in the treatment of DM.


**Keywords:** type 2 diabetes, pharmacogenetics, gene therapy, glucose metabolism, insulin resistance, CRISPR Cas9

## 1. Introduction

According to some sources, diabetes mellitus (DM) is among the oldest human diseases. Diabetes mellitus (DM) is a metabolic condition that is frequently characterized by elevated blood glucose levels that necessitate frequent monitoring and effective control. The hormone insulin is produced by pancreatic beta cells (−cells), which also play a number of other roles in the body. Insulin helps the body's cells absorb glucose for energy

(**Figure 1**). Diabetes mellitus (DM) is brought on by a deficiency in insulin synthesis or sensitivity. It is primarily divided into numerous forms, however type 1 and type 2 DM are the most prevalent types. Type 1 diabetes (T1DM) is characterized by a failure in the pancreatic -cells to produce insulin as a result of T-cell-mediated autoimmunity [1]. Contrarily, type 2 diabetes (T2DM) is characterized by reduced insulin production and insulin resistance. Due to the considerably higher incidence of cardiovascular illnesses and acute metabolic abnormalities in the former group, T1DM was reported to have a shorter life expectancy than T2DM [2]. In order to prevent or delay the development of potential consequences involving other organs such as diabetic nephropathy, retinopathy, neuropathy, cardiovascular illnesses, and diabetic foot ulcers, it is crucial that all kinds of diabetes be recognized and handled at an early stage (**Figure 2a** and **b**) [3–5].

This metabolic condition develops into chronic, life-threatening microvascular, macrovascular, and neuropathic consequences over time. Diabetes mellitus (DM) is brought on by a lack of insulin production, pancreatic cell injury, or insulin resistance brought on by inadequate insulin use. The trend toward sedentary living may be the main cause of the rising number of diabetic patients worldwide, which is predicted to reach 366 million in the older population (>65 years) by 2030 [6]. Nephropathy, neuropathy, cardiovascular and renal issues, retinopathy, food-related diseases, and more are among the many consequences linked to DM.

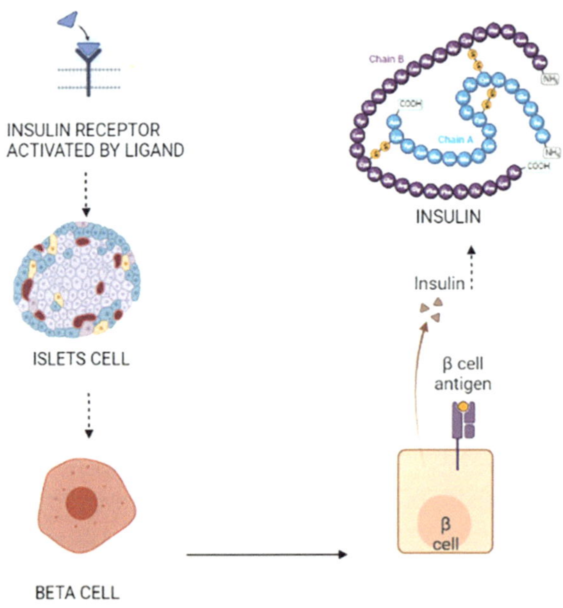


**Figure 1.**
*Insulin receptor gets activated by the binding of ligand, this triggers the islets of Langerhans cells, activating the beta cells (one among four cells types in islets of Langerhans), these produce the hormone insulin and secret them into blood stream. Insulin regulates the activity i.e. the uptake of glucose by the different body organs, tissues and muscles by the action of GLUT4 factor. Any alteration or inhibition in this pathway of glucose production would lead to lack of/or no production of insulin, thus leading to a state of insulin deficiency and further leading to diabetes. If diabetes I s caused by auto immune disfunctioning then its termed as type 1 diabetes and if its caused as a result of insufficient insulin production then it is termed as type 2 diabetes or insulin dependent diabetes.*

*DOI: http://dx.doi.org/10.5772/intechopen.112924*

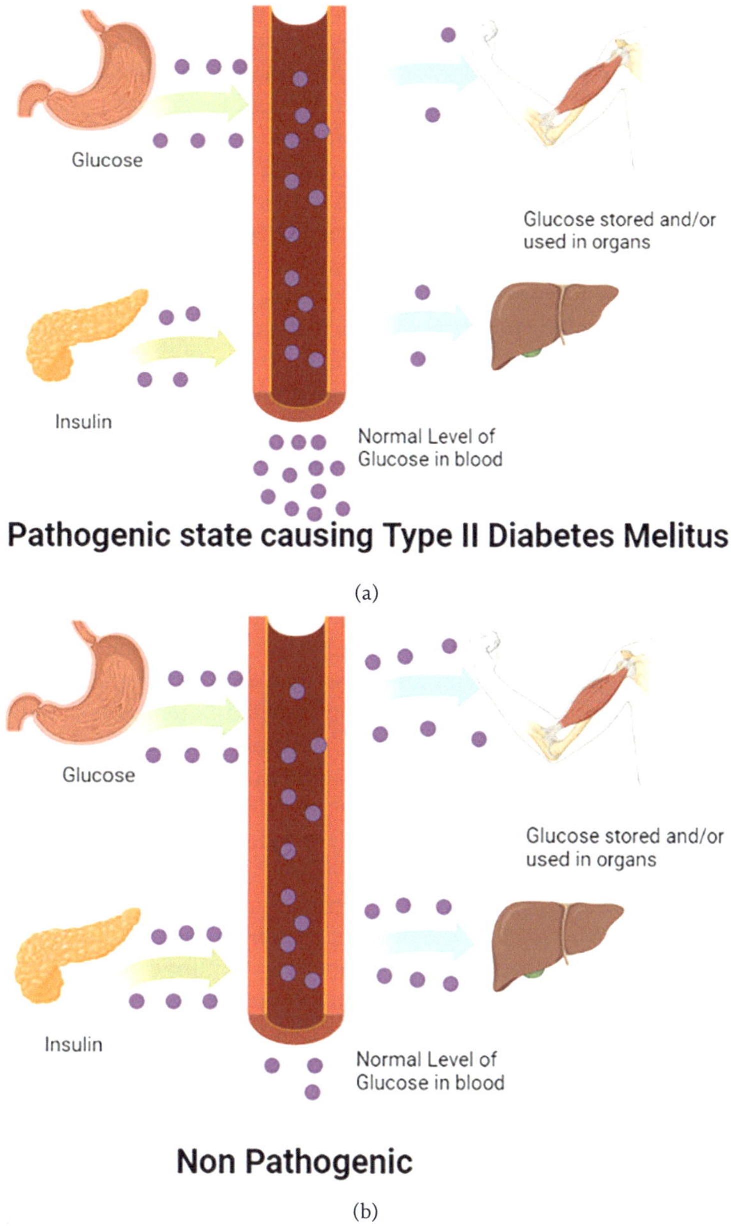


**Figure 2.**
*(a) First image shows a healthy body condition in which pancreatic cells produce enough insulin and thus helping in the adequate glucose intake by organ and other body tissues, this also regulates the blood glucose level, keeping them at normal level. The image shows the glucose being taken up by the organs and also being stored up for further usage, and because of this we see adequate amount of glucose in blood flow and normal blood glucose levels in the body; (b) This figure represents the lack of insulin production and also imbalanced uptake of glucose by the body tissues and organs thus leading to higher concentration of glucose in blood and this condition is referred to as insulin dependent diabetes mellitus. In this the glucose is not adequately absorbed by the cells and organs thus leading to high glucose inflow in blood, eventually leading to increased blood glucose level and also a pathogenic state leading to type II DM.*

Type 2 diabetes (T2D) is a prevalent metabolic disorder characterized by insulin resistance and impaired glucose metabolism. Traditional treatments for T2D have limitations in achieving optimal glucose control and minimizing long-term complications. In recent years, there have been significant advancements in gene therapy that utilize CRISPR-Cas9-mediated gene editing and insulin production, offering potential solutions for the challenges in T2D treatment. The CRISPR-Cas9 technology allows precise modification of specific genes associated with T2D pathogenesis. To ensure effective delivery of the CRISPR-Cas9 complex to target tissues and cells, researchers have explored different methods such as non-viral vectors, viral vectors, and nanocarriers. Moreover, the use of liposomal particles and lecithin nano-liposomal particles as delivery systems enhances the stability and effectiveness of CRISPR-based therapies. These scientific developments hold significant promise in advancing the field of gene therapy for T2D, opening new avenues for personalized and efficacious treatment approaches.

Sulfonylureas, biguiands, peroxisome proliferator activated receptor-, agonists (boosts the action of insulin), and -glucosidase inhibitors (interferes with absorption of glucose in the stomach) are the main conventional types of medications for treating hyperglycemia [7]. These pharmacological types are either used alone or in conjunction with other hypoglycemic medications. The main drawbacks of using the aforementioned conventional drugs include severe hypoglycemia, weight gain, lower therapeutic efficacy due to improper or ineffective dosage regimen, low potency and altered side effects due to drug metabolism and lack of target specificity, solubility and permeability issues [8]. Despite the development of potential anti-hyperglycemic drugs, refining the current therapies to provide optimal and balanced glucose concentrations and lowering long-term consequences from diabetes are the main obstacles to effective diabetes therapy [9]. Type 2 diabetes mellitus (T2DM) is one of the most common metabolic illnesses due to the growth in sedentary behaviors, obesity, and genetic predisposition.

90% of cases of diabetes globally are of type 2, making it the most prevalent type. T2DM is characterized by insulin resistance in peripheral tissues, insulin insufficiency, and poor glucose homeostasis. These factors combine to start a debilitating process that then encourages -cell dysfunction, which further raises morbidity and mortality while decreasing the effectiveness of treatment. Sulphonyurea, meglitinide, biguanide, thiazolidinediones (TZD), and -glucosidase inhibitors are antidiabetic medications. Unfortunately, these therapy approaches are typically limited by gastrointestinal discomfort, weight gain, safety, and tolerability, even when used in combination. The rapid development of genome editing in recent years has boosted human genome research and given researchers a better understanding of the role of single-gene products in the regulation of various disorders [10].

## 2. CRISPR

With several applications in both scientific research and clinical trials, CRISPR has emerged as the most advantageous and effective genome editing technology [11]. There is still potential for improvement even though the use of CRISPR technology for DNA editing has advanced dramatically in recent years. It is challenging and time-consuming to deliver the CRISPR-Cas complex to particular tissues or cells because its components must be delivered into the nucleus for their effect on the nuclear genome to overcome tissue and cell membrane barriers [12]. For the delivery

| Types of species | In vitro/ in vivo | Method of gene delivery | Target gene | Genetic alteration | Types of disease created | Reference |
|---|---|---|---|---|---|---|
| Pig | In vitro | Somatic cell nuclear tRansfer | HTT | Knock in | Huntington | Yan et al. [24] |
| Mouse | In vivo | Stereotactic injection | Ptch1 | Deletion | Medulloblastoma and glioblastoma | Zuckermann et al. [25] |
| New born mice | In vivo | Intravenous infection | OTC | Gene correction | Metabolic liver disease | Yang et al. [26] |
| Rat | In vivo | Subretinal injection | Rho | INDEL mutation | Retinal dystrophy | Bakondi et al. [27] |
| Zebra fish | In vitro | Microinjection | Abcc9,kcnj8 or pln | INDEL mutation | Cardiovascular disease | Tessadori et al. [28] |
| Human | In vitro | Adenoviral transduction | SMAD3 | Gene inactivation | Fibrosis | Voets et al. [29] |

**Table 1.**
*Cellular and animal model of human diseases generated by CRISPR/Cas9.*

of CRISPR-Cas9, non-viral vectors, viral vectors, and physical delivery are frequently used [13, 14]. Electroporation and single-cell microinjection, which are frequently used in embryonic gene editing and the creation of transgenic animals, are the most widely used physical techniques for introducing the CRISPR-Cas complex into cells [15]. Transfer of the Cas DNA or protein components has been done well, with minimal to no cytotoxicity. Microinjection is a laborious and drawn-out procedure that can only be used to deliver the CRISPR-Cas complex to a small number of species [16]. Because they are efficient and effective, particularly for in vivo investigations, viral vectors are frequently utilized as CRISPR-Cas 9 delivery vectors. Given their better cellular uptake and editing potency, viral vectors are currently thought to be the undisputed masters of in vivo CRISPR delivery. Examples of viral delivery vectors include full-sized adenoviruses, lentiviruses, and genetically altered adeno-associated viruses (AAVs). Adeno-associated viral vectors (AAVVs), which have low immunogenicity, cytotoxicity, and limited integration into the host cell, have become the dominant in vivo delivery method for CRISPR components [17]. The lentiviral vector (LV) is another viral vehicle for delivering CRISPR components. It is more effective at cloning than the AAV vector. It can package two copies of an RNA genome (about 10 kilobases), making it a platform for delivering the most common CRISPR/Cas protein (Cas 9) and sgRNA cassette in a single viral transfection event [18]. Due to insertional mutagenesis and the ongoing generation of site-specific nucleases, both of which can result in off-target mutations, LVs present a safe method in therapeutic applications [19]. Scientists have recently created non-integrating lentivirus vectors (NILVs) to deliver CRISPR components in an effort to reduce the risk of integration through either a change in the viral integrase gene or a change in the attachment sequence of lengthy terminal repeats (LTRs) [20]. It is hard to suggest a single viral vector as the best method of delivering CRISPR components because each viral vector has a unique set of advantages and disadvantages. Despite the fact that viral vectors have a high in vivo transfection efficiency, there are substantial problems with their clinical application, such as immunogenicity, integration, and off-target effects. New methods are continually being developed to address these challenges.

Recent studies have shown that using nanocarriers to carry the CRISPR-Cas complex's genes has specific advantages [21]. demonstrates the CRISPR-Cas system's timeframe for use in medicines. The CRISPR-Cas complex has been generated and delivered via a variety of nano-delivery strategies, including cationic liposomes, lipid nanoparticles (LNPs), cationic polymers, vesicles, and gold nanoparticles [14]. Non-viral vectors have emerged as a promising technology in preclinical investigations for the delivery of CRISPR-Cas 9 systems as unique vehicles for extending the application of this technology, hence triggering strong gene-editing in the life sciences and therapeutic settings [22]. As an illustration, cationic arginine gold nanoparticles to transport the Cas 9 protein for causing tumor regression in CC cells by targeting the human AAVS1 gene [23]. Black phosphorus nanosheets (BPs) with Cas 9-RNPs targeting EGFP via cytosolic delivery in a mouse model are used as a biodegradable 2-D delivery platform to elicit tumor regression (**Table 1**) [30].

## 3. CRISPR in diabetes mellitus

There are 463 million instances of diabetes mellitus (DM), a chronic endocrine and metabolic condition with a significant mortality rate, globally [31]. Patients with DM have been treated with insulin, insulin analogs, and non-insulin oral hypoglycemic medications. However, due to inherent pharmacological deficits and restrictions on delivery methods (subcutaneous administration or oral distribution), which led to enzymatic hydrolysis, chemical instability, and subpar gastrointestinal absorption, they were rendered ineffective [32]. A promising therapeutic approach for treating DM is CRISPR gene therapy and nanocarriers, which carry CRISPR to the target locations utilizing liposomes, polymer-based nanoparticles, and inorganic nanoparticles. The CRIPSR can be protected from an enzymatic breakdown in the stomach chambers, improved in vivo stability, and improved bioavailability using nano-carriers. The use of a nanocarrier and the CRISPR-Cas complex reduces the risk of hypoglycemia and boosts patient compliance while replicating endogenous insulin delivery through external stimulation. This treatment can be more focused on specific areas and released gradually over an extended period of time, avoiding adverse effects and maximizing therapeutic effect for the treatment of diabetes [33].

## 4. Treatment of T2DM by lecithin nano-liposomal particle as a CRISPR/Cas9 delivery system

Liposomal particles are great candidate materials given their simple preparation method, easy surface modification, and high biocompatibility. Skyler [34] have recently reported a bio-reducible lipid nanocarrier complex for protein-based Cas9 genome editing. It was produced through electrostatic interaction of cationic lipids and super-negatively charged complexes via protein–protein fusion. Type 2 diabetes mellitus (T2DM) was used as a target disease given its suitability for genetic therapy concerning liver. T2DM is a complex disease characterized by high glucose levels in the bloodstream, reduced glucose processing capacity in adipocytes, and insulin resistance in the body [35]. Elevating glucagon-like peptide-1 (GLP-1), an important target hormone that stimulates insulin secretion, is one of recent therapeutic approaches [36]. However, this hormone has a short half-life due to its extremely rapid degradation by enzyme dipeptidyl peptidase-4 (DPP-4) [37]. To prevent GLP-1 degradation, various drugs inhibiting DPP-4 such as sitagliptin, vildagliptin, saxagliptin, and linagliptin have been developed for insulin-mediated glucose control of T2DM [38]. Moreover, since DPP-4 inhibitors are widely used in clinical practice, they are also investigated as potential new therapeutics against the development of hepatic fibrosis and steatosis [39]. However, small-molecule antidiabetic drugs must be administered daily. In addition, they are associated with adverse effects such as hepatic impairment. T2DM could be treated using a low-risk therapeutic approach such a CRISPR/Cas9-based approach that can efficiently downregulate the DPP-4 enzyme. Cas9-RNP, a ribonucleoprotein made of recombinant Cas9 nuclease complexes and a sgRNA, is intended to modify the DPP-4 gene. A lecithin-based liposomal nanocarrier particle (NL) was created to convey the Cas9-RNP complex. A cationic polymer was included with the Cas9-RNP complex to make up for the negatively charged lipid structure of the NL and boost encapsulation effectiveness. This is so because electrostatic interactions are a major determinant of loading efficiency [40]. Due to the liver's natural metabolism of lecithin, NL are also ideal for addressing liver illnesses from the perspective of biodistribution.

The use of a positively charged polymer improved loading efficiency, which improved Cas9-RNP complex encapsulation. Negatively charged lipids and charge-compensated complexes spontaneously interacted electrostatically, causing NL spheres with a uniform size distribution to self-assemble. The genome platform is ideal for treating genetic and chronic human diseases because it has excellent biocompatibility, low cytotoxicity, and high solution stability, in contrast to unprotected protein therapy techniques that have low delivery efficacy due to enzymatic degradation.

According to the findings, the NL@Cas9-RNP system has a number of benefits, including very effective Cas9-RNP complex encapsulation, efficient and stable in vivo administration, and efficient treatment for liver disease. It is necessary to conduct additional research to characterize and improve the pharmacokinetics, effectiveness, and safety of this DPP-4 gene editing method in animals.

## 5. CRISPR based new tool Cpf1

Recently, a dual-RNA construct known as single guide RNA (sgRNA), which consists of the two components of CRISPR RNA (crRNA) and trans-activating CRISPR RNA (tracrRNA), has been designed by genetic engineering in line with the CRISPR/Cas9 system type II and to ease the usage of this system. When Cas9 binds to tracrRNA, crRNA directs it to the target sequence [41]. This approach relies on RNA rather than protein to assess target specificity, making the technology far more straightforward and accessible. Furthermore, CRISPR/Cas9 is one of the best nuclease-mediated genome editing approaches due to its benefits over meganucleases, ZFNs, and TALENs, including the simplicity of target design, efficiency, and numerous mutations. The Cpf1 family proteins are a group of Cas9 orthologues that were found [42]. These proteins' HNH endonuclease domains are structurally distinct from Cas9's [43]. Technically, the discovery of Cpf1 provided a more straightforward and limited alternative to the CRISPR toolbox by opening up the prospect of more precise genome editing. In terms of its functionality, it belongs to the class of class 2 CRISPR systems. The CRISPR system uses Cpf1 in a different way than Cas9. One RNA molecule would be sufficient to continue the process because, in this case, Cpf1 leaves behind a sticky end rather than a flat one following cleavage (**Figure 3**). Therefore, genes of interest can be consciously

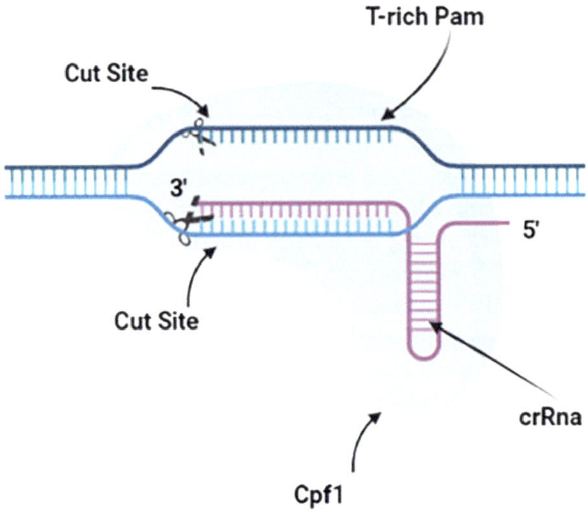


**Figure 3.**
*The CRISPR/Cpf1 technology's molecular processes. Although it differs from CRISPR/Cas9 technically, CRISPR/Cpf1 technology expands the toolkit thanks to its enzyme. Component. A class 2 nuclease, the Cpf1 enzyme exclusively recognizes the target site using one strand of RNA. Based on the location of a T-rich PAM with a TTTN sequence at the 5′ end of crRNA, this enzyme can identify the target sequence. As can be observed, one strand is exactly split at 19 base pairs (bp) after the PAM sequence, and the opposing strand is cleaved at 23 base pairs (bp). When compared to CRISPR/Cas9, the CRISPR/Cpf1 sticky ends boost the specificity and functional efficiency.*

put into vectors utilizing CRISPR/Cpf1 technology. Because of this, Cpf1 is more effective than Cas9 [44]. Cpf1 circumvents HDR's efficiency restriction for genome editing in non-diverging cells [45]. The CRISPR/Cas9 system can only target sites with PAMs with NGG sequences, which restricts gene editing at target sites with G-rich sequences. Cpf1 fixes this issue in the interim by identifying the T-rich target locations. The other benefit of Cpf1 over Cas9 is the ability to target a greater variety of places in the genome thanks to the addition of this option to the gene editing toolbox. Researchers recently created Cpf1 proteins that include uridine-rich 3′ ends in addition to a complementary 20-bp target site to increase the efficacy of Cpf1 in inducing INDEL mutations in target locations [46].

## 6. CRISPR Cas9 treatment using CLAN nano-particle-

Although the NLRP3 inflammasome is a well-researched target for the therapy of a number of auto-inflammatory illnesses, including diabetes, there is still much to be done. Using a cationic lipid-Nano-carrier to deliver CRISPR-Cas9 into macrophages for the downregulation of NLRP3 via CLAN encapsulated mCas9 and gRNA-targeting NLRP3 in macrophages is a potential method for treating NLRP3-dependent DM. This increases insulin vulnerability and decreases inflammation in the adipose tissue of type 2 diabetes caused by high-fat diets (HFDs) by inhibiting the activation of the NLRP3 inflammasome to minimize acute inflammation post-intravenous injection [47].

Another study used a library of cationic lipid-assisted PEG-b-PLGA nanoparticles (CLAN) with varying polymer compositions (PEG5K-b-PLGA11K, PLGA8K, and cationic lipid BHEM-Chol), surface density, and surface charges to deliver the

CRISPR-Cas9 system to neutrophils in the epididymal white adipose tissue and liver [47]. Similar to this, macrophage-specific CRISPR-Cas9 plasmids targeting Ntn1 gene encased in cationic lipid-assisted PEG-b-PLGA nanoparticles (CLAN) via intravenous injection have been shown to decrease Ntn1 gene expression and improve Type 2 diabetes (T2D) symptoms both in vitro and in vivo [48]. Based on the aforementioned research, it can be deduced that the precision delivery of the CRISPR-Cas9 system to the Ntn1, elastase, NLRP3, and DPP4 genes to produce Type 2 DM regression is aided by cationic and lipid nanoparticles. To learn more about their molecular process, however, additional research in the animal model is required.

## 7. Islet amyloid polypeptide (IAPP) and T2DM

Islet amyloid polypeptide (IAPP, amylin), a polypeptide hormone of [49] amino acid residues that is released by islet beta cells [50], was identified, isolated, and given the name from islet tumor cells. Under the influence of glucose and other secretagogues, it is mostly deposited in the halo of the secretory granule and secreted in pulses [51]. IAPP creates oligomers that lead to beta cell death and so promote islet amyloidosis. In short, IAPP produces oligomers that lead to beta cell death and promote islet amyloidosis, which in turn cause insulin secretion to gradually fail [52]. The main function of IAPP in the process of glucose metabolism is to block the manufacture of glycogen, the transit of glucose, the uptake of glucose by muscle tissue, and the use of glucose by hepatocytes [53]. The single subunit state of the soluble IAPP protein is unfolded. In order to more accurately control human blood sugar, it can work in synergy with hormones that control blood glucose, such as insulin [54]. The mature human IAPP protein (hIAPP) can form amyloid aggregates and has a strong propensity to misfold. Of the 20 amyloid aggregated peptides that have been found so far, hIAPP is one of the most heavily aggregated polypeptides [55]. According to several investigations, islet amyloid deposition was discovered in the islets of people with type 2 diabetes. Amyloidosis of the hIAPP is seen as a potentially.

Since pigs are biologically the most similar to humans than any other species, they were chosen to serve as the model for this HiAPP protein study. This protein's expression and analysis were studied to determine its impact on T2DM using a CRISPR Cas9-based gene editing technology.

## 8. Conclusion

In conclusion, this literature provides a comprehensive overview of the advancements in gene therapy for type 2 diabetes using CRISPR-Cas9-mediated gene editing and insulin production. The introduction highlights the significance of diabetes mellitus (DM) as a chronic metabolic condition and the limitations of conventional medications in achieving optimal glucose control and minimizing long-term consequences. The abstract delves into the advancements in CRISPR technology, discussing various delivery methods for the CRISPR-Cas complex, including non-viral vectors, viral vectors, and nanocarriers. It also explores the potential of CRISPR gene therapy and nanocarriers in treating DM, targeting specific factors such as the NLRP3 inflammasome and the DPP-4 enzyme. Liposomal particles and lecithin nano-liposomal particles are discussed as efficient delivery systems for CRISPR/Cas9, with potential applications in treating type 2 diabetes. The role of islet amyloid polypeptide (IAPP) in type 2 diabetes and its study using CRISPR-Cas9-based gene editing technology is also presented. The treatment of type 2 diabetes using CRISPR technology holds great promise for overcoming the limitations of current therapies. The use of CRISPR-Cas9 and nanocarriers provides advantages such as improved stability, targeted delivery, and prolonged release of therapeutic agents. Non-viral vectors, viral vectors, and physical delivery methods have been explored for delivering the CRISPR-Cas complex to specific tissues or cells. Each method has its advantages and limitations, and ongoing research aims to address the challenges associated with clinical applications. The application of CRISPR technology in type 2 diabetes involves targeting specific genes or factors involved in the disease process. The downregulation of the NLRP3 inflammasome and DPP-4 enzyme using CRISPR gene therapy and nanocarriers shows promise in improving insulin sensitivity, reducing inflammation, and enhancing glucose control. The use of liposomal particles and lecithin nano-liposomal particles as CRISPR/Cas9 delivery systems has demonstrated efficient encapsulation and targeted delivery to the liver, a relevant organ in type 2 diabetes management. Furthermore, the study of islet amyloid polypeptide (IAPP) using CRISPR-Cas9-based gene editing technology provides insights into the role of this peptide in glucose metabolism and its potential contribution to beta cell dysfunction. By understanding the mechanisms underlying IAPP aggregation and its impact on insulin secretion, researchers can develop innovative strategies for managing type 2 diabetes. Overall, the advancements in CRISPR technology offer exciting possibilities for the treatment of type 2 diabetes. The use of gene editing and nano-carriers can improve the effectiveness and specificity of therapeutic interventions, potentially leading to better glucose control, reduced complications, and improved quality of life for individuals with type 2 diabetes. Further research and development in this field are needed to optimize delivery methods, ensure safety and efficacy, and translate these advancements into clinical practice. The discovery and development of novel therapies, including those derived from natural products, in combination with CRISPR technology, hold great promise for the future of diabetes treatment.

## Author details

Sairam Venkatraman, Srinivasan S. Tharun, Ashok Pavithra and Reddy Amala*
Department of Biotechnology, School of Bioengineering, SRM Institute of Science and Technology (SRMIST), Kattankulathur, Tamil Nadu, India

*Address all correspondence to: amalar@srmist.edu.in

## References

[1] Gharravi AM, Jafar A, Ebrahimi M, Mahmodi A, Pourhashemi E, Haseli N, et al. Current status of stem cell therapy, scaffolds for the treatment of diabetes mellitus. Diabetes and Metabolic Syndrome: Clinical Research & Reviews. 2018;**12**:1133-1139

[2] Wise J. Type 1 diabetes is still linked to lower life expectancy. BMJ. 2016;**1**:2

[3] Khalil H. Diabetes microvascular complications—a clinical update. Diabetes and Metabolic Syndrome: Clinical Research & Reviews. 2017;**11**:S133-S139

[4] Papatheodorou K, Papanas N, Banach M, Papazoglou D, Edmonds M. Complications of diabetes. Journal Diabetes Research. 2016;**2016**:1-3

[5] Ahmad J. The diabetic foot. Diabetes and Metabolic Syndrome: Clinical Research & Reviews. 2016;**10**:48-60

[6] Wild S, Roglic G, Green A, Sicree R, King H. Global prevalence of diabetes: Estimates for the year 2000 and projections for 2030 diabetes. Care. 2004;**27**:1047-1053. DOI: 10.2337/diacare.27.5.1047

[7] Chaudhury A, Duvoor C, Dendi VSR, Kraleti S, Chada A, Ravilla R, et al. Clinical review of antidiabetic drugs: Implications for type 2 diabetes mellitus management. Frontiers in Endocrinology. 2017;**8**:1-12. DOI: 10.3389/fendo.2017.00006

[8] Feingold KR, Anawalt B, Boyce A, editors. Oral and Injectable (Non-insulin) Pharmacological Agents for Type 2 Diabetes. South Dartmouth (MA): MDText.com, Inc; 2000 Available from: https://www.ncbi.nlm.nih.gov/books/NBK279141/

[9] Li H, Yang Y, Hong W, Huang M, Wu M, Zhao X. Applications of genome editing technology in the targeted therapy of human diseases: Mechanisms, advances and prospects. Signal Transduct Target Therapy. 2020;**5**:1

[10] Bhattacharjee R, Nandi A, Mitra P, Saha K, Patel P, Jha E, et al. Theragnostic application of nanoparticle and CRISPR against food-borne multi-drug resistant pathogens. Materials Today Biotechnology. 2022;**15**:4

[11] Glass Z, Lee M, Li Y, Xu Q. Engineering the delivery system for CRISPR-based genome editing. Trends in Biotechnology. 2018;**36**:173-185

[12] Behr M, Zhou J, Xu B, Zhang H. In vivo delivery of CRISPR-Cas9 therapeutics: Progress and challenges. Acta Pharma Sinica B. 2021;**11**:2150-2171

[13] Nath A, Bhattacharjee R, Nandi A, Sinha A, Kar S, Manoharan N, et al. Phage delivered CRISPR-Cas system to combat multidrug-resistant pathogens in gut microbiome. Biomedicine & Pharmacotherapy. 2022;**151**:4

[14] Horodecka K, Düchler M. Crispr/cas9: Principle, applications, and delivery through extracellular vesicles. International Journal of Molecular Sciences. 2021;**22**:5

[15] Duan L, Ouyang K, Xu X, Xu L, Wen C, Zhou X, et al. Nanoparticle delivery of CRISPR/Cas9 for genome editing. Frontiers in Genetics. 2021;**12**:4

[16] Verdera HC, Kuranda K, Mingozzi F. Vector immunogenicity in humans: A long journey to successful gene transfer. Molecular Therapy. 2020;**28**:723-746

[17] Yi BH. Recent advances in CRISPR/Cas9 delivery strategies. Biomolecules. 2020;**10**:4

[18] Bushman FD. Retroviral insertional mutagenesis in humans: Evidence for four genetic mechanisms promoting expansion of cell clones. Molecular Therapy. 2020;**28**:352-356

[19] Gurumoorthy N, Nordin F, Tye GJ, Zaman WSWK, Ng MH. Non-integrating lentiviral vectors in clinical applications: A glance through. Biomedicine. 2022;**10**:4

[20] Deng H, Huang W, Zhang Z. Nanotechnology based CRISPR/Cas9 system delivery for genome editing: Progress and prospect. Nano Research. 2019;**12**:2437-2450

[21] Rabiee N, Bagherzadeh M, Ghadiri AM, Fatahi Y, Aldhaher A, Makvandi P, et al. Turning toxic nanomaterials into a safe and bioactive nanocarrier for co-delivery of DOX/pCRISPR. ACS Applied Bio Materials. 2021;**4**:5336-5351

[22] Mout R, Ray M, Yesilbag Tonga G, Lee YW, Tay T, Sasaki K, et al. Direct cytosolic delivery of CRISPR/Cas9-ribonucleoprotein for efficient gene editing. ACS Nano. 2017;**11**:2452-2458

[23] Zhou W, Cui H, Ying L, Yu X-F. Enhanced cytosolic delivery and release of CRISPR/Cas9 by black phosphorus nanosheets for genome editing. Angewandte Chemie. 2018;**130**:10425-10429

[24] Zuckermann M, Hovestadt V, Knobbe-Thomsen CB, et al. Somatic CRISPR/Cas9-mediated tumour suppressor disruption enables versatile brain tumour modelling. Nature Communications. 2015;**6**:7391

[25] Yang Y, Wang L, Bell P, et al. A dual AAV system enables the Cas9-mediated correction of a metabolic liver disease in newborn mice. Nature Biotechnology. 2016;**34**(3):334

[26] Bakondi B, Lv W, Lu B, et al. In vivo CRISPR/Cas9 gene editing corrects retinal dystrophy in the S334ter-3 rat model of autosomal dominant retinitis pigmentosa. Molecular Therapy. 2016;**24**:556-563

[27] Iuchi S, Kuldell N. Zinc Finger Proteins: From Atomic Contact to Cellular Function. USA: Springer Science & Business Media; 2007

[28] Voets O, Tielen F, Elstak E, et al. Highly efficient gene inactivation by adenoviral CRISPR/Cas9 in human primary cells. PLoS One. 2017;**12**(8):e0182974

[29] Zinman B et al. Empagliflozin: Cardiovascular outcomes, and mortality in type 2 diabetes. The New England Journal of Medicine. 2015;**373**(22):2117-2128

[30] Charpentier E, Richter H, van der Oost J, White MF. Biogenesis pathways of RNA guides in archaeal and bacterial CRISPR-Cas adaptive immunity. FEMS Microbiology Reviews. 2015;**39**:428-441

[31] Wang A, Yang T, Fan W, Yang Y, Zhu Q, Guo S, et al. Protein corona liposomes achieve efficient oral insulin delivery by overcoming mucus and epithelial barriers. Advanced Healthcare Materials. 2019;**8**:5

[32] Cho EY, Ryu JY, Lee HAR, Hong SH, Park HS, Hong KS, et al. Lecithin nano-liposomal particle as a CRISPR/Cas9 complex delivery system for treating type 2 diabetes. Journal of Nanobiotechnology. 2019;**17**:5

[33] Xu C, Lu Z, Luo Y, Liu Y, Cao Z, Shen S, et al. Targeting of NLRP3 inflammasome with gene editing for the amelioration of inflammatory diseases. Nature Communication. 2018;**9**:6

[34] Skyler JS. Diabetes mellitus: Pathogenesis and treatment strategies. Journal of Medicinal Chemistry. 2004;**47**:4113-4117

[35] Baggio LL, Drucker DJ. Biology of incretins: GLP-1 and GIP. Gastroenterology. 2007;**132**:2131-2157

[36] Drucker DJ, Nauck MA. The incretin system: Glucagon-like peptide-1 receptor agonists and dipeptidyl peptidase-4 inhibitors in type 2 diabetes. Lancet. 2006;**368**:1696-1705

[37] Rohrborn D, Wronkowitz N, Eckel J. DPP-4 in diabetes. Frontiers in Immunology. 2015;**6**:386

[38] Scheen AJ. Pharmacokinetic and toxicological considerations for the treatment of diabetes in patients with liver disease. Expert Opinion on Drug Metabolism & Toxicology. 2014;**10**:839-857

[39] Pohl C, Kiel JA, Driessen AJ, Bovenberg RA, Nygard Y. CRISPR/Cas9 based genome editing of penicillium chrysogenum. ACS Synthetic Biology. 2016;**5**:754-764

[40] Brender JR et al. Amyloid fiber formation and membrane disruption are separate processes localized in two distinct regions of IAPP, the type-2- diabetes-related peptide. Journal of the American Chemical Society. 2008;**130**:6424-6429

[41] Zetsche B, Gootenberg JS, Abudayyeh OO, et al. Cpf1 is a single RNA-guided endonuclease of a class 2 CRISPR-Cas system. Cell. 2015;**163**:759-771

[42] Makarova KS, Wolf YI, Alkhnbashi OS, et al. An updated evolutionary classification of CRISPR–Cas systems. Nature Reviews. Microbiology. 2015;**13**:722-736

[43] Li T, Zhu L, Xiao B, Gong Z, Liao Q, Guo J. CRISPR-Cpf1-mediated genome editing and gene regulation in human cells. Biotechnology Advances. 2019;**37**:21-27

[44] Nami F, Basiri M, Satarian L, Curtiss C, Baharvand H, Verfaillie C. Strategies for in vivo genome editing in nondividing cells. Trends in Biotechnology. 2018;**36**:770-786

[45] Moon SB, Lee JM, Kang JG, et al. Highly efficient genome editing by CRISPR-Cpf1 using CRISPR RNA with a uridinylate-rich 3′-overhang. Nature Communications. 2018;**9**:3651

[46] Sena CM, Bento CF, Pereira P, Marques F, Seiça R. Diabetes Mellitus: New Challenges and Innovative Therapies. Springer EMPA. 2013:29-87. DOI: 10.1007%2Fs13167-010-0010-9

[47] Luo YL, Xu CF, Li HJ, Cao ZT, Liu J, Wang JL, et al. Macrophage-specific in vivo gene editing using cationic lipid-assisted polymeric nanoparticles. ACS Nano. 2018;**12**:994-1005

[48] Wang M, Zuris JA, Meng F, Rees H, Sun S, Deng P, et al. Efficient delivery of genome-editing proteins using bioreducible lipid nanoparticles. Proceedings of the National Academy Science USA. 2016;**113**:2868-2873

[49] Kahn SE et al. Evidence of cosecretion of islet amyloid polypeptide and insulin by β-cells. Diabetes. 1990;**39**:634-638

[50] Marzban L, Trigo-Gonzalez G, Verchere CB. Processing of pro-islet

amyloid polypeptide in the constitutive and regulated secretory pathways of β cells. Molecular Endocrinology. 2005;**19**:2154-2163

[51] Pithadia A, Brender JR, Fierke CA, Ramamoorthy A. Inhibition of IAPP aggregation and toxicity by natural products and derivatives. Journal Diabetes Research. 2016;**2016**:12

[52] Grimm J, Heitz F, Wirth F, Welt T. Novel compounds capable of antagonizing islet amyloid polypeptide (iapp) induced beta-cell damage and impaired glucose tolerance. Google Patents. 2018

[53] Chiti F, Dobson CM. Protein misfolding, amyloid formation, and human disease: A summary of progress over the last decade. Annual Review of Biochemistry. 2017;**86**:27-68

[54] Camargo DCR et al. The redox environment triggers conformational changes and aggregation of hIAPP in type II diabetes. Scientific Reports. 2017;7:44041

[55] Mukherjee A, Morales-Scheihing D, Butler PC, Soto C. Type 2 diabetes as a protein misfolding disease. Trends in Molecular Medicine. 2015;**21**:439-449

Chapter 4

# Impact of Pharmacogenetics Markers of Human *NAT2* Gene in Tuberculosis Treatment

*Victória Moraes-Silva, Cecilia Alvim Dutra, Márcia Quinhones P. Lopes, Philip Noel Suffys, Adalberto Rezende Santos, Harrison Magdinier Gomes and Raquel Lima de F. Teixeira*

## Abstract

Tuberculosis (TB), mainly caused by *Mycobacterium tuberculosis*, accounts for 10 million cases worldwide per year, remaining a major problem for public health. The anti-TB drug isoniazid (INH) is recommended by the WHO. Despite of effective drugs, some individuals do not respond to standard treatment that can result in varying degrees of adverse drug reactions. One of the factors related to the variability in individual response to treatment is the presence of polymorphisms in genes encoding drug-metabolizing proteins, which can alter the protein's activity. The *NAT2* gene encodes Arylamine N-acetyltransferase 2 (NAT2), the main enzyme responsible for INH metabolism. Genetic variants found in *NAT2* coding region affect N-acetylation. The rate of substrate metabolism defines the phenotype of individuals as fast, intermediate, slow, or ultra-slow acetylators. The slow phenotype has been associated with high risk of hepatotoxicity during TB treatment, and this risk is shown to be greater when an ultra-slow acetylator is identified. Furthermore, fast phenotype could be associated with extensive TB treatment due to greater drug clearance and therefore lower bioavailability of INH. The identification and use of biomarkers for phenotype prediction could minimize unfavorable therapeutic outcomes and optimize the effectiveness of tuberculosis treatment.

**Keywords:** tuberculosis, pharmacogenetics, N-acetyltransferase 2, NAT2, isoniazid

## 1. Introduction

Tuberculosis (TB) disease is mainly caused by *Mycobacterium tuberculosis*, and it is estimated that about a quarter of the world's population is infected by this bacterium. Out of this total, approximately 10% will develop active tuberculosis, while the remaining 90% will have noncommunicable tuberculosis. According to data published by the WHO in 2022 for the previous year, it is estimated that 10.6 million people fell ill with tuberculosis in 2021, resulting in 1.6 million deaths worldwide. These numbers highlight the prevalence of cases in low- and middle-income countries accounting for 98% of reported TB. TB is the 13th leading cause of death globally and ranks first in deaths caused by a single infectious agent with only COVID-19 in 2020 (surpassing HIV/AIDS) having higher numbers. Thus, TB remains a major health problem for the world population. In 2021, according to WHO data, TB cases are distributed as follows: Southeast Asia (45%), Africa (23%), Western Pacific (18%), Eastern Mediterranean (8.1%), Americas (2.9%), and Europe (2.2%). Thirty countries with the highest TB burden accounted for 87% of all estimated incidence cases worldwide, and eight of these countries contribute to two-thirds of the global total: India (28%), China (7.4%), Indonesia (9.2%), the Philippines (7.0%), Pakistan (5.8%), Nigeria (4.4%), Bangladesh (3.6%), and Democratic Republic of the Congo (2.9%) [1]. The estimated TB incidence rates for 2021 can be observed in **Figure 1**.

Isoniazid (INH) [2], rifampicin (RIF) [3], pyrazinamide (PZA) [4], and ethambutol [5] (EMB) are the four antibiotics indicated as first-line treatment for TB. The standard TB treatment comprises a first phase with isoniazid, rifampicin, pyrazinamide, and ethambutol, for 2 months with fixed dosages, followed by a second phase that includes the use of only INH and RIF for an additional 4 months. The first 2 months of TB treatment are responsible for killing of metabolically active and dormant bacilli, and most of the sputum smear-positive patients turn negative within this period [3, 4]. Traditionally, the prescription of standard fixed-dose (FDC) combination drugs has been recommended to simplify and facilitate treatment and adherence. These combinations of four drugs have some advantages, such as cost-effectiveness and universal access, low relapse rate (estimated at 3–5%), and intermittent administration in most cases.

Although the standard 6-month treatment regimen is highly effective for drug-susceptible *Mycobacterium tuberculosis*, some limitations are related to TB treatment, such as long duration, access to treatment in low- and middle-income country with limited financial capacity, and adverse drug reactions (ADRs). The most common ADRs associated with INH are peripheral neuropathy and hepatotoxicity, while reactions with an unestablished frequency include nausea, vomiting, stomach pain, fever, lymphadenopathy, skin rash, and vasculitis [2]. For RIF, ADRs include nausea, vomiting, and hepatitis, whereas the frequency of hyperbilirubinemia and cholestasis has

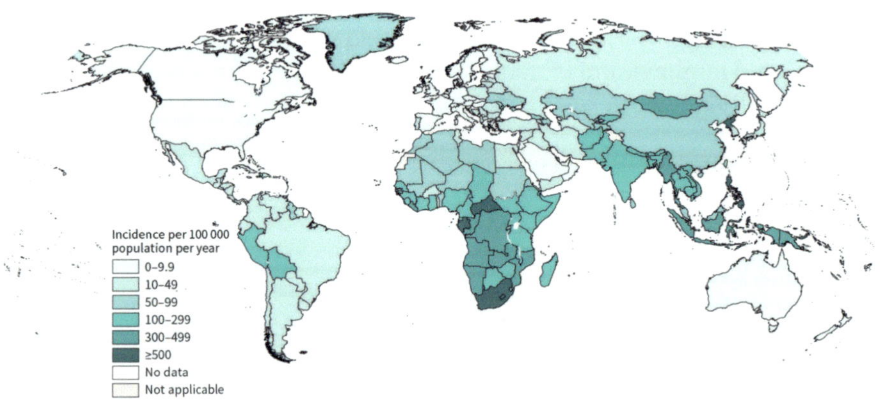


**Figure 1.**
*Estimated TB incidence rates, 2021 [1].*

not been established [3]. One severe ADR, life-threatening liver injury (about 14%), is related to the use of 3 g daily of PZA, while arthralgia, vomiting, anorexia, general malaise, sideroblastic anemia, urticaria, and increased uric acid were not frequency determined [4]. Finally, optic neuritis is the most frequent ADR related to EMB, followed by arthralgia, abdominal discomfort or pain, malaise, headache, vertigo, and mental confusion with undetermined frequency [5].

The antituberculosis drug-induced liver injury (ATDILI) affects from 2 to 28% of patients treated with multidrug therapy for TB and is potentially serious and fatal, leading to treatment interruption and failure [6].

Individuals on the same therapeutic regimen show a variability in their response. ADRs are one of the main causes of morbidity and mortality in developed countries, affecting both children and adults. Additionally, they have a negative socioeconomic impact, leading to hospitalizations and prolonged treatment times. Several factors contribute to this variability, including age, sex, nutritional status, general medical condition, lifestyle, concomitant therapy, presence of comorbidity, and genetic factors. The genetic background of individuals can play a significant role in determining the outcomes of TB treatment [7].

Variations in the human genome sequence, such as single-nucleotide polymorphisms (SNPs), involve a replacement of one nucleotide base with any one of the other three, occurring at approximately once every 1000 bases in the human genome. When SNPs are located on genes encoding metabolic enzymes, transport proteins, or cell surface receptors, they may affect the pharmacokinetics (PK—absorption, distribution, metabolism, excretion) and pharmacodynamics (PD—drug-target interaction and dose-effect relationship) of the drug. Pharmacogenetics can be defined as the branch of pharmacology that studies how variations influence drug response and its effects. Pharmacogenomics is an innovative approach aimed at minimizing ADRs and maximizing treatment effectiveness.

The significant differences in individuals' drug responses are evident, considering that it is estimated that individuals differ from each other every 300–1000 nucleotides, resulting in approximately 10 million SNPs. Identifying which of these variants or combinations of variants have functional consequences for long-term drug effects will be enable the development individualized therapy based on the patient's genetic sequence, leading to an adequate response and prevention adverse reactions [8–11].

Certain genes are correlated with the pharmacokinetics and pharmacodynamics of drugs used for TB treatment, such as *NAT2*, *CYP2E1*, *GSTT1*, *GSTM1*, and *SLCO*. When these genes encode proteins with low activity, there is a higher incidence of hepatitis (**Table 1**).

Isoniazid is a prodrug that requires activation by the catalase/peroxidase enzyme (KatG) of *M. tuberculosis*, resulting in the production of reactive oxygen radicals (superoxide, hydrogen peroxide, and peroxynitrate) and organic radicals. These radicals inhibit the formation of mycolic acid in the bacterial cell wall, causing damage to the DNA and subsequent death of the bacillus. The most common mechanism of resistance to isoniazid involves mutations in katG, which decrease its activity, preventing the conversion of the prodrug into its active metabolite. Isoniazid is considered a primary drug and is used in the treatment of all forms of tuberculosis caused by strains of *M. tuberculosis* that are sensitive to it. Its biotransformation occurs in the liver through acetylation. In humans, there is genetic heterogeneity in the rate of isoniazid acetylation and liver disease may prolong the clearance of isoniazid. It inhibits the synthesis of mycolic acid, an important component of the wall of mycobacteria, not acting against other types of bacteria.

| Drug | Gene | Allele | Nucleotide Change(s)/rs Identifiers | Amino Acid Change(s) | Protein Function | Risk Phenotype | Reference |
|---|---|---|---|---|---|---|---|
| Isoniazid | *NAT2* | *NAT2*6* | c.590G > A (rs1799930) | R197Q | Slow | Slow acetylation | [12, 13] |
| | | *NAT2*7* | c.857G > A (rs1799931) | G286E | Slow | | [12, 14] |
| | | *NAT2*14* | c.191G > A (rs1801279) | R64Q | Slow | | [12, 15, 16] |
| | *CYP2E1* | *CYP2E1*1A* | −1053 C > T | — | Slow | Slow detoxification | [17, 18] |
| | | *CYP2E1*5* | -1293G > C | — | Slow | | [17, 18] |
| | *GST* | *GSTM1*0* | null genotype | — | Absence | Slow detoxification | [18] |
| | | *GSTT1*0* | null genotype | — | Absence | | [19] |
| Rifampicin | *SLCO1B1* | *SLCO1B1*5* | c.521 T > C (rs4149056) | V174A | Slow | Decreased Transport | [20] |
| | | *SLCO1B1*37* | c.388A > G (rs2306283) | N130D | Slow | | [21] |
| | | *SLCO1B1*4* | c.463C > A (rs11045819) | P155T | Slow | | [22] |
| | | *SLCO1B1*15* | c.50611A > G (rs2306283)<br>c.52422 T > C (rs4149056) | N130D V174A | Slow | | [23] |
| | *ABCB1* | — | c. 3435C > T (rs1045642) | I1145I (synonymous) | Slow | Decreased Transport | [24] |
| | | — | c.2677G > T (rs2032582) | S893A | Slow | | [24] |
| | | — | c.1236C > T (rs1128503) | G412G (synonymous) | Slow | | [24] |

*ND: not determined.*

**Table 1.**
*Association of genetic variants with risk of liver damage induced by anti-tuberculosis drugs.*

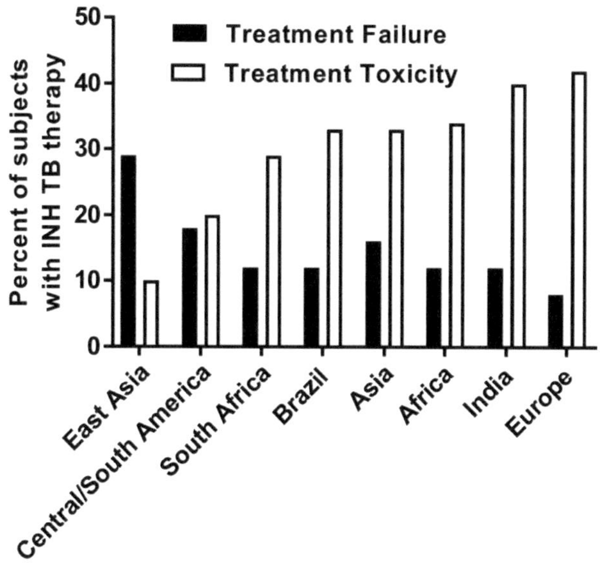


**Figure 2.**
*Estimated frequency of therapeutic failure and treatment toxicity with INH for tuberculosis in populations worldwide [12]. Adapted from [28].*

Isoniazid (INH) is metabolized in the liver *via* N-acetyltransferase (NAT2) generating acetylhydrazine; when oxidized by cytochrome P4502E1 (CYP2E1), it can form hepatotoxic intermediates [25, 26]. Another route of INH metabolism is direct hydrolysis to hydrazine, a potent hepatotoxin. These reactive metabolites can destroy hepatocytes by interfering with cellular homeostasis or triggering immune reactions in which reactive metabolites bound to plasma proteins in hepatocytes can act as haptens [27]. **Figure 2** shows the estimated frequency of therapeutic failure and treatment toxicity with INH for tuberculosis in populations worldwide. Standard TB therapy, including INH, results in more than 40% of patients experiencing ADR and more than 30% with treatment failure in populations around the world. Therefore, pharmacogenomics-guided therapy is highly cost-effective and directly impacts INH-induced liver injury and treatment response [28].

## 2. N-acetyltransferase 2

Human N-acetyltransferase 2 is a phase II biotransformation enzyme predominantly expressed in the liver, small intestine, and colon [29]. NAT2 was first identified in humans in 1960 and is a 33.79 kDa [30] cytosolic enzyme with the role of catalyzing N-acetylation and O-acetylation, through the transfer of the acetyl group from the acetyl-Coenzyme A (acetyl-CoA) cofactor to the nitrogen terminal of hydrazines, arylamines, and heterocyclic amines [31, 32]. NAT2 is involved in the metabolism and inactivation of substances that include carcinogens and drugs used in the treatment of infections and chronic diseases, such as tuberculosis, leprosy, and arterial hypertension, among others [32, 33].

The high-resolution structure of human NAT2 was determined by Wu et al. [31] and defines three protein domains. The first, named as the N-terminal domain, comprises residues 1–83 and consists of five helices and a short β strand present between α2 and α3 helices. The second domain, comprising residues 84–192, is composed of nine β strands and two short helices. These two domains are connected to the third domain, called C-terminal (residues 230–290), through the α-helical interdomain (residues 193–229; helices α8– α10), which is composed of four antiparallel β strands and one helix [31]. The catalytic triad, located in the N-terminal domain of the protein structure, consists of three highly conserved residues: cysteyne at position 68, Histidine 107, and aspartic acid 122. Their interaction occurs through the donation of the acetyl group of the acetyl-CoA cofactor to a sulfhydryl residue of the catalytic site cysteine, forming acetylcysteinyl as an intermediate structure. Subsequently, the acetyl group is transferred to the amino terminus of the substrate [34–36].

The molecular study of human N-acetyltransferases revealed two homologous genes, encoding *NAT1* and *NAT2*, and a pseudogene, *pNAT* [37]. These loci are located on chromosome 8 (8p22). N-acetyltransferase 2 is encoded by *NAT2,* an intronless gene that has 873 bp [38]. SNPs in the *NAT2* gene-coding region can alter enzymatic activity, resulting in three different phenotypes: fast acetylators (FAs) with two functional alleles, intermediate acetylators with one functional allele combined with a "slow" allele, and slow acetylators (SAs) with two "slow" alleles [39]. According to the official NAT2 nomenclature website, the arylamine N-acetyltransferases (NATs) database (http://nat.mbg.duth.gr/) [40], more than 100 SNPs and 108 haplotypes have been identified. The reference *NAT2*4* allele was first identified in the Japanese population and does not have any SNP in its coding region The protein encoded by *NAT2*4* confers FA phenotype [13, 41, 42]. The *NAT2* alleles or haplotypes are characterized by the combination of up to six simultaneous SNPs. They are commonly clustered into specific allelic groups based on signature SNP: haplotypes belonging to the *NAT2*5* allelic group share the c.341 T > C, SNP signature just as the *NAT2*6* allelic group share the c.590G > A, SNP signature. The c.857G > A SNP characterizes *NAT2*7* cluster, and c.191C > A is common for *NAT2*14* alleles [43]. The frequencies of *NAT2* allelic groups among different populations can be seen in **Table 2**.

Mutations can cause various effects on the activity and function of a protein through four main mechanisms: decreased mRNA levels, altered protein levels, altered protein stability, and direct alteration of protein activity [43]. Although SNPs can influence NAT2 activity, it is essential to consider the haplotype to fully understand the genotype-phenotype relationship. Previous studies of enzymatic activity with the most frequent *NAT2* alleles/haplotypes have enabled the characterization of the acetylation profile, making them potential biomarkers for enhancing therapeutic treatment or preventing the increase of the number of cancer cases. However, understanding the prior genotypic profile of the population is required [43].

SNPs discovery studies of the *NAT2* gene have been performed in diverse populations. Among the seven SNPs commonly found in *NAT2* (**Table 3**), four (c.191G > A/ rs1801279, c.341 T > C/rs1801280, c.590G > A/ rs1799930, and c.857G > A/ rs1041983) are non-synonymous mutations that result in a significant decrease in acetylation capacity, and the other three (c.282C > T/ rs1799929, c.481C > T/ rs1799931, and c.803A > G/rs1208) are synonymous SNPs or do not change the acetylation phenotype [11, 13, 39, 55]. There are 13 *NAT2* haplotypes; eight of them are widely distributed, with three associated with rapid acetylation phenotype (*NAT2**4, *NAT2**12A, and *NAT2**13A), and the other five are related to slow acetylation phenotypes (*NAT2**5B, *NAT2**6A, *NAT2**7B, *NAT2**5C, and *NAT2**5A) [56].

| Population (N) | *NAT2* haplotypes, % (2 N = 100%) | | | | | | | Reference |
|---|---|---|---|---|---|---|---|---|
| | *4 | *5 | *6 | *7 | *12 | *13 | *14 | |
| America | | | | | | | | |
| Brazilian (404) | 20 | 38 | 27 | 4 | 4 | 3 | 4 | [44] |
| Ngawbe (105) | 72.4 | 2.4 | 0 | 23.3 | 0 | 1.9 | ND | [45] |
| Embera (136) | 61 | 9.9 | 3.7 | 22.8 | 0 | 2.6 | ND | [45] |
| Africa | | | | | | | | |
| Tswana (101) | 13.4 | 32.2 | 20 | 0 | 20.8 | 6.4 | 8.4 | [46] |
| Mandenka (97) | 9.3 | 36.1 | 17 | 6.7 | 15.5 | 5.2 | 10.3 | [47] |
| Sudanese (127) | 8.7 | 47.2 | 28.7 | 3.1 | 8.3 | 0.8 | 3.1 | [48] |
| Europe | | | | | | | | |
| Spanish (1312) | 22.2 | 45.7 | 26.7 | 1.2 | 2.6 | 0.3 | 1.4 | [49] |
| German (844) | 22.7 | 46.5 | 27.8 | 1.3 | ND | 1.5 | 0.1 | [50] |
| US Caucasian (387) | 24.2 | 45.9 | 26.6 | 1.9 | 0.4 | 0.9 | 0.1 | [51] |
| Russian (364) | 23.5 | 45.6 | 27.2 | 3.2 | 0.5 | 0 | 0 | [52] |
| Asia | | | | | | | | |
| Chinese (212) | 59.2 | 4 | 20.8 | 14.9 | 0.7 | 0.5 | 0 | [53] |
| Japanese (200) | 69.5 | 0.5 | 19.8 | 8.8 | ND | 1.3 | ND | [54] |

*ND: not determined.*

**Table 2.**
*Frequencies of NAT2 allelic groups among populations worldwide.*

| SNP | rs Identifiers | Amino Acid Change(s) | Protein Function | Reference |
|---|---|---|---|---|
| c.191G > A | rs1801279 | R64Q | Slow | [13, 39] |
| c.282C > T | rs1799929 | Y94Y (synonymous) | Rapid | [13, 39] |
| c.341 T > C | rs1801280 | I114T | Slow | [13, 39] |
| c.481C > T | rs1799931 | L161L (synonymous) | Rapid | [13, 39] |
| c.590G > A | rs1799930 | R197Q | Slow | [13, 39] |
| c.803A > G | rs1208 | K268R | Rapid | [13, 39] |
| c.857G > A | rs1041983 | G286E | Slow | [13, 39] |

**Table 3.**
*The seven SNPs commonly found in NAT2.*

The identification of the mutation frequency allows a virtual pre-definition of the phenotypic profile in a closed ethnic population. African populations exhibit the highest level of diversity within a population, characterized by a low frequency of the *NAT2*4* haplotype but a high frequency of the other two fast haplotypes, *NAT2*12A* and *NAT2*13A*. In fact, *NAT2*12A* is called the hallmark of this population, as it is rarely found outside Africa. However, this population also has a high frequency of slow acetylator alleles. In European populations, the *NAT2*5B* and *NAT2*6A* haplotypes, associated with the slow acetylation phenotype, are predominant over the fast *NAT2*4* haplotype. Descendants of European and sub-Saharan Africans with slow acetylator genotypes represent about 50% of the population [56].

In relation to Asia, characterized by one of the highest frequencies of *NAT2*4* in the world (**Table 2**) and a low diversity of haplotypes, only three other alleles occur with frequency > 0.01: *NAT2*6A*, *NAT2*7B*, and *NAT2*14*, which confer a low acetylation protein [11, 56]. On the other hand, the American continent has a high level of population diversity, like the African population, indicating remarkable heterogeneity for *NAT2* variation in this region [56]. The difference found can be easily explained by the presence of several small populations isolated as a result of the displacement of people over the years from larger populations, including those with European and African ancestry. This explains the presence of the *NAT2*6A*, *NAT2*7B*, and *NAT2*14* haplotypes in this region [26]. In Brazilians, an admixture population, some studies have shown the high allelic diversity of *NAT2*, including the description of new or rare SNPs and alleles (*NAT2*5O*, **6 M* and **12E*) with unknown functional effect [11, 55]. The high frequency of slow acetylators found in the Brazilian population may be related to the high rate of miscegenation between the European (colonizer) and African (slave) populations [55].

Several studies have shown that low activity of NAT2 enzymes can significantly impact drug treatment of individuals and pose risks. Recently, two independent studies have further refined the low enzymatic activity in slow acetylators and ultraslow acetylators, and their heterogeneity was observed when comparing genotypes of the same classification. The difference in heterogeneity is measured through the Odds Ratio (OR), which represents the chance of an event occurring in a group or between groups. Specific *NAT2*5* genotypes (c.341 T > C), *NAT2*6* (c.590G > A), *NAT2*7* (c.857G > A), and *NAT2*14* (c.191G > A) show amino acid substitutions in the protein (I114T, R197Q, G286E, and R64Q, respectively) [57, 58]. This sub-characterization of the markers allows to the identification of risks associated with each cluster/haplotype, enabling better therapeutic targeting and reanalysis of the literature, which might have overlooked data with a lower risk of occurrence of the class.

Literature data have demonstrated the great importance of functional knowledge of N-acetylation for patients treated with anti-TB drugs such as INH. The slow acetylation state contributes to the occurrence of hepatotoxicity (adverse hepatic effects) during TB treatment, characterized by liver damage caused by excessive ingestion of chemicals or risk of antituberculosis drug-induced liver injury (ATDILI), defined by an increase of more than twice in the upper limit of normal value (ULN) in alanine transaminase (ALT) or aspartate aminotransferase (AST) and long-term bilirubin [55, 59, 60].

Individuals carrying the genotype *NAT2*4/*5* and *NAT2**4/*6 exhibit similar acetylation values. However, when the wild-type allele is absent, the variant alleles *NAT2*5* and *NAT2*6* confer different acetylation capacities [56]. A gene dose effect can be observed for these variant alleles within slow acetylation phenotype, as there is a statistically significant trend toward slower than expected acetylation capability when genotypes are combined: *NAT2*5/*5* > *NAT2*5/*6* > *NAT2*6/*6*. *NAT2*6/*6* shows a reduction of almost 30% in their enzymatic activity compared to the *NAT2*5/*5* homozygote [61].

Comparing individuals with a high-activity enzyme to slow acetylators, Teixeira et al. in 2011 observed a 2.8-fold increased risk of ATDILI occurrence (95% CI:

2.20–3.57; P = 5.73E − 18) for the slow acetylation genotype [11]. Meanwhile, while Suvichapanich *et al. in* 2018 observed that the ultraslow subgroups (based on combined genotypes *6A/*6A, *6A/*7B, and *7B/*7B) were able to achieve a 3.6-fold increased risk (95% CI: 2, 30–5.63; P = 1.76E −08) of ATDILI. Furthermore, N-acetylation enzymatic kinetics assays with recombinant human NAT2 demonstrated that the activity of NAT2*4 was 7.6–22-fold greater than that of NAT*5 and *6, respectively. Additionally, the Vmax/Km value of NAT2*5B was 3.2 and 4.7 times higher than those of *6A and *7B, respectively, indicating better catalytic efficiency when compared to other low-activity alloenzymes [57]. Therefore, it is evident that ultraslow acetylators may contribute to a higher risk of ATDILI than other classes [61].

It is believed that in INH metabolism, the decrease in NAT activity can alter the elimination of hydrazine and N-acetylhydrazine, leading individuals with these genotypes to be exposed to hepatotoxins for a longer time, increasing susceptibility to ATDILI. Additionally, ATDILI occurrence may be due to the redirection of INH pharmacological metabolism to hydrolysis, a minor pathway that results in a greater amount of hydrazine, given the decreased NAT activity [62].

The pharmacokinetic variability caused by the diverse distribution of polymorphisms in NAT2 has posed a challenge for implementing a standard dosage of INH. While the relationship between the slow acetylation profile and the occurrence of adverse reactions is clear, the relationship between the fast acetylation profile, inadequate serum levels of INH, and the occurrence of unfavorable outcomes is not well understood, with conflicting results in the main studies. Fast acetylators are characterized by the absence of SNPs in the *NAT2* coding region or by the presence of variants that do not affect N-acetylation, such as c.282C > T, c.481 > T, c.803A > G, and c.845A > C or a combination of some of them (*NAT2*11A*, *NAT*12A*, *NAT2*12B*, *NAT2*12C*, *NAT2*13A*, and *NAT2*18* alleles) [15, 40, 50, 63–65].

According to Peloquin *et al.* [66], fast acetylators have a clearance rate of isoniazid 1.4 and 3.6 times higher than intermediate and slow acetylators, respectively. This results in faster drug elimination and less absorption, leading to lower exposure to INH than what is considered effective. Fast acetylators are more likely to present a positive sputum culture after 2 months of treatment [66, 67]. A prolonged therapeutic response may have consequences such as extended treatment time, low patient adherence, and higher financial cost, due to possible hospitalizations and greater demand for medication. Additionally, the drug may not reach the minimum concentration necessary to be effective against the bacilli, potentially leading to the selection of resistant strains [67, 68].

According to Jing *et al.* [69], even with the administration of a high dose of INH (900 mg/day), only 66.1% of the patients with fast acetylation reached the maximum concentration. However, when using the standard dosage (300 mg/day), more than 98% of fast acetylators, 89.1% of intermediate acetylators, and only 26.9% of slow acetylators achieved Cmax values lower than the minimum recommended dose (3 μg/mL) [69]. These findings show that the standard used INH dosages used for intermediate and fast acetylators are insufficient, and adjusting the INH dose based on NAT2 metabolism status may be necessary to achieve an improved balance between risk and benefit during treatment.

Pharmacokinetic assays have been increasingly incorporated into clinical routine, especially in the developed countries, with the aim of proposing appropriate dosages for new drugs. Studies conducted in Asia and the United States have demonstrated significant differences in INH clearance based on different acetylation phenotypes [62, 66]. Moreover, the variations in acetylation profiles among different populations underscore the variable influence of NAT2 polymorphisms, emphasizing the importance of genotypic identification before administering isoniazid [69]. Pharmacogenetic research involves candidate genes that can function as biomarkers associated with drug metabolism and transport, enabling the prediction of drug toxicity and efficacy.

## 3. Conclusions

According to the model proposed by Russmann et al. [70], several factors may be responsible for the variability of the therapeutic response, such as nongenetic factors (age, sex, nutritional status, general medical condition, lifestyle, concomitant therapy, or presence of comorbidity, etc.) and genetic factors. Among them are the SNPs that when located in genes encoding metabolic enzymes, transporters, or receptors, may be able to change pharmacokinetics and pharmacodynamics of the drug [70].

An important study tool is pharmacogenetics that could be used to identify variants in the *NAT2* gene. This characterization allows for the prediction of possible therapeutic outcomes unwanted in TB treatment. According to the data obtained, it was possible to visualize that slow acetylators are more likely to develop adverse effects than fast acetylators. Besides, it is important to refine the phenotype prediction in subcategories, to identify the "ultraslow" acetylators and analyze the real risk for this subcategory.

The NAT2 slow acetylator and the risk of antituberculosis drug-induced liver injury (ATDILI) is confirmed. Among them, the recently proposed subgroup of ultraslow acetylators stands out, with patients with *NAT2* genotypes of *6A/*6A, *6A/*7B, and *7B/*7B, contributing to an increased risk of ATDILI (OR: 3.60; 95% CI: 2.30–5.63; P = 1.76E − 08) than all NAT2 slow acetylators (OR: 2.80; 95% CI: 2.20–3.57; P = 5.73E − 18), as well as fast acetylators [61].

It is known that the acquisition of drug resistance is related not only to the pathogen but also to the host. It was observed that in certain populations with high rates of therapeutic failure and acquisition of bacterial resistance, patients under anti-TB treatment had lower-than-expected serum drug levels, mostly fast acetylators [66, 71].

The study set of studies in relation to pharmacogenomics diagnosis, the effect on clinical outcomes, and patient development for everyday clinical use should be developed. Accumulated data on NAT2 clinical significance support the replacement as non-weighted standard therapy practices with pharmacogenomics-guided therapies. Thus, researchers look for factors that justify the development of new approaches to direct the treatment of tuberculosis, such as, the use of pharmacogenomics for NAT2. This practice will benefit treatment by reducing adverse effects and increasing efficiency [13, 41].

## Acknowledgements

To the support of the research team involved in this work, and to the support of Oswaldo Cruz Foundation/IOC and funding from CAPES.

## Author details

Victória Moraes-Silva, Cecilia Alvim Dutra, Márcia Quinhones P. Lopes, Philip Noel Suffys, Adalberto Rezende Santos, Harrison Magdinier Gomes and Raquel Lima de F. Teixeira*
Laboratory of Molecular Biology Applied to Mycobacteria –Oswaldo Cruz Institute – Fiocruz, Rio de Janeiro, RJ, Brazil

*Address all correspondence to: ft.raquel@gmail.com

## References


[1] Word Health Organization (WHO). Global tuberculosis report 2021. Geneva: WHO; 2021. Available from: https://www.who.int/teams/global-tuberculosis-programme/tb-reports/global-tuberculosis-report-2022

[2] Zhang Y. The magic bullets and tuberculosis drug targets. Annual Review of Pharmacology and Toxicology. 2005;**45**:529-564. DOI: 10.1146/annurev.pharmtox.45.120403.100120

[3] Blumberg HM, Burman WJ, Chaisson RE, Daley CL, Etkind SC, Friedman LN, et al. American Thoracic Society/Centers for Disease Control and Prevention/Infectious Diseases Society of America: Treatment of tuberculosis. American Journal of Respiratory and Critical Care Medicine. 2003;**167**(4):603-662. DOI: 10.1164/rccm.167.4.603

[4] Zhang Y, Yew WW. Mechanisms of drug resistance in mycobacterium tuberculosis. The International Journal of Tuberculosis and Lung Disease. 2009;**13**(11):1320-1330. Available from: https://www.ingentaconnect.com/content/iuatld/ijtld/2009/00000013/00000011/art00004;jsessionid=2s5a7bd9sxlvl.x-ic-live-03#

[5] Handbook of anti-tuberculosis agents. Introduction. Tuberculosis (Edinburgh, Scotland). 2008;**88**(2):85-86. DOI: 10.1016/S1472-9792(08)70002-7

[6] Tostmann A, Boeree MJ, Aarnoutse RE, de Lange WC, van der Ven AJ, Dekhuijzen R. Antituberculosis drug-induced hepatotoxicity: Concise up-to-date review. Journal of Gastroenterology and Hepatology. 2008;**23**:192-202. DOI: 10.1111/j.1440-1746.2007.05207.x

[7] Resende LS, Santos-Neto ET. Risk factors associated with adverse reactions to antituberculosis drugs. Jornal Brasileiro de Pneumologia. 2015;**41**(1):77-89. DOI: 10.1590/S1806-37132015000100010

[8] Relling MV, Giacomini KM. Pharmacogenetics. In: Brunton LL, Lazo GS, Parker KL, editors. Goodman & Gilman's : The Pharmacological Basis of Therapeutics. XI edizione ed. New York: McGraw-Hill Medical Publishing Division; 2006, Chapter 4. pp. 93-115

[9] Bachtiar M, Ooi BNS, Wang J, et al. Towards precision medicine: Interrogating the human genome to identify drug pathways associated with potentially functional, population-differentiated polymorphisms. The Pharmacogenomics Journal. 2019;**19**(06):516-527. DOI: 10.1038/s41397-019-0096-y

[10] Barbarino JM, Whirl-Carrillo M, Altman RB, Klein TE. PharmGKB: A worldwide resource for pharmacogenomic information. Wiley Interdisciplinary Reviews. Systems Biology and Medicine. 2018;**10**(04):e1417. DOI: 10.1002/wsbm.1417

[11] Teixeira RLF, Morato RG, Cabello PH, Muniz LMK, Moreira ASR, Kritski AL, et al. Genetic polymorphisms of NAT2, CYP2E1 and GST enzymes and theoccurrence of antituberculosis drug-induced hepatitis in Brazilian TB patients. MemInst Oswaldo Cruz. 2011;**106**:716-724. DOI: 10.1590/S0074-02762011000600011

[12] Hein DW, Millner LM. Arylamine N-acetyltransferase acetylation polymorphisms: Paradigm for pharmacogenomic-guided therapy- A focused review. Expert

Opinion on Drug Metabolism and Toxicology. 2021;**17**(1):9-21. DOI: 10.1080/17425255.2021.1840551

[13] Fretland AJ, Leff MA, Doll MA, Hein DW. Functional characterization of human N-acetyltransferase 2 (NAT2) single nucleotide polymorphisms. Pharmacogenetics. 2001;**11**(3):207-215. DOI: 10.1097/00008571-200104000-00004

[14] Blum M, Demierre A, Grant DM, Heim M, Meyer UA. Molecular mechanism of slow acetylation of drugs and carcinogens in humans. Proceedings of the National Academy of Sciences of the United States of America. 1991;**88**(12):5237-5241. DOI: 10.1073/pnas.88.12.5237

[15] Hein DW, Ferguson RJ, Doll MA, Rustan TD, Gray K. Molecular genetics of human polymorphic N-acetyltransferase: Enzymatic analysis of 15 recombinant wild-type, mutant, and chimeric NAT2 allozymes. Human Molecular Genetics. 1994;**3**(5):729-734. DOI: 10.1093/hmg/3.5.729

[16] Huang YS, Chern HD, Su WJ, Wu JC, Lai SL, Yang SY, et al. Polymorphism of the N-acetyltransferase 2 gene as a susceptibility risk factor antituberculosis drug-induced hepatitis. Hepatology. 2002;**35**:883-889. DOI: 10.1053/jhep.2002.32102

[17] Vuilleumier N, Rossier MF, Chiappe A, Degoumois F, Dayer P, Mermillod B, et al. CYP2E1 genotype and isoniazid-induced hepatotoxicity in patients treated for latent tuberculosis. European Journal of Clinical Pharmacology. 2006;**62**(6):423-429. DOI: 10.1007/s00228-006-0111-5

[18] Huang YS. Genetic polymorphisms of drug-metabolizing enzymes and the susceptibility to antituberculosis drug-induced liver injury. Expert Opinion on Drug Metabolism & Toxicology. 2007;**3**(1):1-8. DOI: 10.1517/17425255.3.1.1

[19] Leiro V, Fernández-Villar A, Valverde D, Constenla L, Vázquez R, Piñeiro L, et al. Influence of glutathione S-transferase M1 and T1 homozygous null mutations on the risk of antituberculosis drug-induced hepatotoxicity in a Caucasian population. Liver International. 2008;**28**(6):835-839. DOI: 10.1111/j.1478-3231.2008.01700.x

[20] Nozawa T, Imai K, Nezu J, Tsuji A, Tamai I. Functional characterization of pH-sensitive organic anion transporting polypeptide OATP-B in human. The Journal of Pharmacology and Experimental Therapeutics. 2004;**308**(2):438-445. DOI: 10.1124/jpet.103.060194

[21] Chen R, Wang J, Tang S, Zhang Y, Lv X, Wu S, et al. Association of polymorphisms in drug transporter genes (SLCO1B1 and SLC10A1) and anti-tuberculosis drug-induced hepatotoxicity in a Chinese cohort. Tuberculosis (Edinburgh, Scotland). 2015;**95**(1):68-74. DOI: 10.1016/j.tube.2014.11.004

[22] Tirona RG, Leake BF, Merino G, Kim RB. Polymorphisms in OATP-C: Identification of multiple allelic variants associated with altered transport activity among European- and African-Americans. The Journal of Biological Chemistry. 2001;**276**(38):35669-35675. DOI: 10.1074/jbc.M103792200

[23] Niemi M, Schaeffeler E, Lang T, Fromm MF, Neuvonen M, Kyrklund C, et al. High plasma pravastatin concentrations are associated with single nucleotide polymorphisms and haplotypes of organic anion transporting polypeptide-C (OATP-C, SLCO1B1). Pharmacogenetics.

2004;**14**(7):429-440. DOI: 10.1097/01.fpc.0000114750.08559.32

[24] Fung KL, Gottesman MM. A synonymous polymorphism in a common MDR1 (ABCB1) haplotype shapes protein function. Biochimica et Biophysica Acta. 2009;**1794**(5):860-871. DOI: 10.1016/j.bbapap.2009.02.014

[25] Nelson SD, Mitchell JR, Timbrell JA, Snodgrass WR, Corcoran GB 3rd. Isoniazid and iproniazid: Activation of metabolites to toxic intermediates in man and rat. Science. 1976;**193**(4256):901-903. DOI: 10.1126/science.7838

[26] Timbrell JA, Mitchell JR, Snodgrass WR, Nelson SD. Isoniazid hepatotoxicity: The relationship between covalent binding and metabolism in vivo. The Journal of Pharmacology and Experimental Therapeutics. 1980;**213**:364-369. DOI: 10022-3565/80/2132.0364$02.OO/O2.00/0

[27] Lee WM. Drug-induced hepatotoxicity. The New England Journal of Medicine. 2003;**349**(5):474-485. DOI: 10.1056/NEJMra021844

[28] Rens NE, Uyl-de Groot CA, Goldhaber-Fiebert JD, et al. Costeffectiveness of a pharmacogenomic test for stratified isoniazid dosing in treatment of active tuberculosis. Clinical Infectious Diseases. 2020;**71**(12): 3136-3143. DOI: 10.1093/cid/ciz1212

[29] Evans DA, Manley KA, McKusick VA. Genetic control of isoniazid metabolism in man. British Medical Journal. 1960;**2**(5197):485-491. DOI: 10.1136/bmj.2.5197.485

[30] Evans DA. N-acetyltransferase. Pharmacology & Therapeutics. 1989;**42**(2):157-234. DOI: 10.1016/0163-7258(89)90036-3

[31] Wu H, Dombrovsky L, Tempel W, Martin F, Loppnau P, Goodfellow GH, et al. Structural basis of substrate-binding specificity of human arylamine N-acetyltransferases. The Journal of Biological Chemistry. 2007;**282**(41):30189-30197. DOI: 10.1074/jbc.M704138200. Epub 2007 Jul 26

[32] Rajasekaran M, Abirami S, Chen C. Effects of single nucleotide polymorphisms on human N-acetyltransferase 2 structure and dynamics by molecular dynamics simulation. PLoS One. 2011;**6**(9):e25801

[33] Husain A, Zhang X, Doll MA, States JC, Barker DF, Hein DW. Identification of N-acetyltransferase 2 (NAT2) transcription start sites and quantitation of NAT2-specific mRNA in human tissues. Drug Metabolism and Disposition. 2007;**35**(5):721-727. DOI: 10.1124/dmd.106.014621

[34] Dupret JM, Grant DM. Site-directed mutagenesis of recombinant human arylamine N-acetyltransferase expressed in Escherichia coli. Evidence for direct involvement of Cys68 in the catalytic mechanism of polymorphic human NAT2. Journal of Biological Chemistry. 1992;**267**(11):7381-7385. DOI: 10.1016/S0021-9258(18)42528-8

[35] Rodrigues-Lima F, Dupret JM. 3D model of human Arylamine N-acetyltransferase 2: Structural basis of variant R64Q slow Acetylator phenotype and active site loop analysis. Biochemical and Biophysical Research Communications. 2002;**291**(1):116-123. DOI: 10.1006/bbrc.2002.641

[36] Wang H, Vath GM, Gleason KJ, Hanna PE, Wagner CR. Probing the mechanism of hamster arylamine N-acetyltransferase 2 acetylation by active site modification, site-directed mutagenesis, and pre-steady state and

steady state kinetic studies. Biochemistry. 2004;**43**(25):8234-8246. DOI: 10.1021/bi0497244

[37] García-Martín E. Interethnic and intraethnic variability of NAT2 single nucleotide polymorphisms. Current Drug Metabolism. 2008;**9**(6):487-497. DOI: 10.2174/138920008784892155

[38] Sachidanandam R, Weissman D, Schmidt SC, Kakol JM, Stein LD, Marth G, et al. A map of human genome sequence variation containing 1.42 million single nucleotide polymorphisms. Nature. 2001;**409**(6822):928-933. DOI: 10.1038/35057149

[39] Hein DW. Genética molecular e função de NAT1 e NAT2: papel no metabolismo de aminasaromáticas e carcinogênese. Mutation Research. 2002;**506-507**:65-77. DOI: 10.1016/s0027-5107(02)00153-7

[40] Bisso-Machado R, Ramallo V, Paixão-Côrtes VR, Acuña-Alonzo V, Demarchi DA, Sandoval JR, et al. NAT2 gene diversityand its evolutionarytrajectory in the Americas. The Pharmacogenomics Journal. 2016;**16**(6):559-565. DOI: 10.1038/tpj.2015.72

[41] Zang Y, Doll MA, Zhao S, States JC, Hein DW. Functional characterizatin of single-nucleotide polymorphisms and haplotypes of human N-acetyltransferase 2. Carcinogenesis. 2007;**28**(8):1665-1671. DOI: 10.1093/carcin/bgm085

[42] Sabbagh A, Darlu P, Crouau-Roy B, Poloni ES. Arylamine N-acetyltransferase 2 (NAT2) genetic diversity and traditional subsistence: A worldwide population survey. PLoS One. 2011;**6**(4):e18507. DOI: 10.1371/journal.pone.0018507

[43] Walraven JM, Zang Y, Trent JO, Hein DW. Structure/function evaluations of single nucleotide polymorphisms in human N-acetyltransferase 2. Current Drug Metabolism. 2008;**9**(6):471-486. DOI: 10.2174/138920008784892065

[44] Teixeira RL, Miranda AB, Pacheco AG, Lopes MQ, Fonseca-Costa J, Rabahi MF, et al. Genetic profile of thearylamine N-acetyltransferase 2 coding gene among individuals from two different regions of Brazil. Mutation Research. 2007;**624**(1-2):31-40. DOI: 10.1016/j.mrfmmm.2007.03.015

[45] Jorge-Nebert LF, Eichelbaum M, Griese EU, Inaba T, Arias TD. Analysis of six SNPs of NAT2 in Ngawbe and Embera Amerindians of Panama and determination of the Embera acetylation phenotype using caffeine. Pharmacogenetics. 2002;**12**(1):39-48. DOI: 10.1097/00008571-200201000-00006

[46] Loktionov A, Moore W, Spencer SP, Vorster H, Nell T, O'Neill IK, etal.DifferencesinN-acetylationgenotypes between Caucasians and black south Africans: Implications for cancer prevention. Cancer Detection and Prevention. 2002;**26**(1):15-22. DOI: 10.1016/s0361-090x(02)00010-7

[47] Sabbagh A, Langaney A, Darlu P, Gérard N, Krishnamoorthy R, Poloni ES. Worldwide distribution of NAT2 diversity: Implications for NAT2 evolutionary history. BMC Genetics. 2008;**9**:21. DOI: 10.1186/1471-2156-9-21

[48] Al-Yahyaee S, Gaffar U, Al-Ameri MM, Qureshi M, Zadjali F, Ali BH, et al. N-acetyltransferase polymorphism among northern Sudanese. Human Biology. 2007;**79**(4):445-452. DOI: 10.1353/hub.2007.0047

[49] Agúndez JA, Golka K, Martínez C, Selinski S, Blaszkewicz M, García-Martín E. Unraveling ambiguous NAT2 genotyping data. Clinical Chemistry. 2008;**54**(8):1390-1394. DOI: 10.1373/clinchem.2008.105569

[50] Cascorbi I, Drakoulis N, Brockmöller J, Maurer A, Sperling K, Roots I. Arylamine N-acetyltransferase (NAT2) mutations and their allelic linkage in unrelated Caucasian individuals: Correlation with phenotypic activity. American Journal of Human Genetics. 1995;**57**(3):581-592

[51] Deitz AC, Zheng W, Leff MA, Gross M, Wen WQ, Doll MA, et al. N-Acetyltransferase-2 genetic polymorphism, well-done meat intake, and breast cancer risk among postmenopausal women. Cancer Epidemiology, Biomarkers & Prevention. 2000;**9**(9):905-910

[52] Belogubova EV, Kuligina ES, Togo AV, Karpova MB, Ulibina JM, Shutkin VA, et al. 'Comparison of extremes' approach provides evidence against the modifying role of NAT2 polymorphism in lung cancer susceptibility. Cancer Letters. 2005;**221**(2):177-183. DOI: 10.1016/j.canlet.2004.11.008

[53] Song DK, Xing DL, Zhang LR, Li ZX, Liu J, Qiao BP. Association of NAT2, GSTM1, GSTT1, CYP2A6, and CYP2A13 gene polymorphisms with susceptibility and clinicopathologic characteristics of bladder cancer in Central China. Cancer Detection and Prevention. 2009;**32**(5-6):416-423. DOI: 10.1016/j.cdp.2009.02.003

[54] Machida H, Tsukamoto K, Wen CY, Shikuwa S, Isomoto H, Mizuta Y, et al. Crohn's disease in Japanese is associated with a SNP-haplotype of N-acetyltransferase 2 gene. World Journal of Gastroenterology. 2005;**11**(31):4833-4837. DOI: 10.3748/wjg.v11.i31.4833

[55] Ruiz JD, Martínez C, Anderson K, Gross M, Lang NP, García-Martín E, et al. The differential effect of NAT2 variant alleles permits refinement in phenotype inference and identifies a very slow acetylation genotype. PLoS One. 2012;**7**:44629. DOI: 10.1371/journal.pone.0044629

[56] Selinski S, Blaszkewicz M, Ickstadt K, Hengstler JG, Golka K. Refinement of the prediction of N-acetyltransferase 2 (NAT2) phenotypes with respect to enzyme activity and urinary bladder cancer risk. Archives of Toxicology. 2013;**87**(12):2129-2139. DOI: 10.1007/s00204-013-1157-7

[57] Suvichapanich S, Fukunaga K, Zahroh H, et al. NAT2 ultra-slow acetylator and risk of anti-tuberculosis drug-induced liver injury: A genotype-based meta-analysis. Pharmacogenetics and Genomics. 2018;**28**(7):167-176. DOI: 10.1097/FPC.000000000 0000339

[58] Scales MD, Timbrell JA. Studies on hydrazine hepatotoxicity 1. : Pathologica findings. Journal of Toxicology and Environmental Health. 1982;**10**:941-953. DOI: 10.1080/15287398209530308

[59] Azuma J, Ohno M, Kubota R, Yokota S, Nagai T, Tsuyuguchi K, et al. NAT2 genotype guided regimen reduces isoniazid-induced liver injury and early treatment failure in the 6-month four-drug standard treatment of tuberculosis: A randomized controlled trial for pharmacogenetics-based therapy. European Journal of Clinical Pharmacology. 2013;**69**(5):1091-1101. DOI: 10.1007/s00228-012-1429-9

[60] Mah A, Kharrat H, Ahmed R, Gao Z, Der E, Hansen E, et al. Serum drug concentrations of INH and RMP

predict 2-month sputum culture results in tuberculosis patients. The International Journal of Tuberculosis and Lung Disease. 2015;**19**(2):210-215. DOI: 10.5588/ijtld.14.0405

[61] Pasipanodya JG, McIlleron H, Burger A, Wash PA, Smith P, Gumbo T. Serum drug concentrations predictive of pulmonary tuberculosis outcomes. The Journal of Infectious Diseases. 2013;**208**(9):1464-1473. DOI: 10.1093/infdis/jit352

[62] Seng KY, Hee KH, Soon GH, Chew N, Khoo SH, Lee LS. Population pharmacokinetic analysis of isoniazid, acetylisoniazid, and isonicotinic acid in healthy volunteers. Antimicrobial Agents and Chemotherapy. 2015;**59**(11):6791-6799. DOI: 10.1128/AAC.01244-15. Epub 2015 Aug 17

[63] Peloquin CA. Therapeutic drug monitoring in the treatment of tuberculosis. Drugs. 2002;**62**(15):2169-2183. DOI: 10.2165/00003495-200262150-00001

[64] Sekine A, Saito S, Iida A, Mitsunobu Y, Higuchi S, Harigae S, et al. Identification of single-nucleotide polymorphisms (SNPs) of human N-acetyltransferase genes NAT1, NAT2, AANAT, ARD1 and L1CAM in the Japanese population. Journal of Human Genetics. 2001;**46**(6):314-319. DOI: 10.1007/s100380170065

[65] Lin HJ, Han CY, Lin BK, Hardy S. Ethnic distribution of slow acetylator mutations in the polymorphic N-acetyltransferase (NAT2) gene. Pharmacogenetics. 1994;**4**(3):125-134. DOI:10.1097/00008571-199406000-00003

[66] Peloquin CA, Jaresko GS, Yong CL, Keung AC, Bulpitt AE, Jelliffe RW. Population pharmacokinetic modeling of isoniazid, rifampin, and pyrazinamide. Antimicrobial Agents and Chemotherapy. 1997;**41**(12):2670-2679. DOI: 10.1128/AAC.41.12.2670

[67] Jung JA, Kim TE, Lee H, Jeong BH, Park HY, Jeon K, et al. A proposal for an individualized pharmacogenetic-guided isoniazid dosage regimen for patients with tuberculosis. Drug Design, Development and Therapy. 2015;**9**:5433-5438. DOI: 10.2147/DDDT.S87131

[68] Ungcharoen U, Sriplung H, Mahasirimongkol S, Chusri S, Wichukchinda N, Mokmued P, et al. The influence of NAT2 genotypes on isoniazid plasma concentration of pulmonary tuberculosis patients in southern Thailand. Tuberculosis and Respiratory Diseases (Seoul). 2020;**83**(Supple 1):S55-S62

[69] Jing W, Zong Z, Tang B, Wang J, Zhang T, Wen S, et al. Population pharmacokinetic analysis of isoniazid among pulmonary tuberculosis patients from China. Antimicrobial Agents and Chemotherapy. 2020;**64**(3):e01736-e01719, /aac/64/3/AAC.01736-19.atom. DOI: 10.1128/AAC.01736-19

[70] Russmann S, Kullak-Ublick GA, Grattagliano I. Current concepts of mechanisms in drug-induced hepatotoxicity. Current Medicinal Chemistry. 2009;**16**(23):3041-3053. DOI: 10.2174/092986709788803097

[71] Ray J, Gardiner I, Marriott D. Managing antituberculosis drug therapy by therapeutic drug monitoring of rifampicin and isoniazid. Internal Medicine Journal. 2003;**33**(5-6):229-234. DOI: 10.1046/j.1445-5994.2003.00390.x

Chapter 5

# Pharmacogenomics of Cardiovascular Diseases: The Path to Precision Therapy

*Georges Nemer and Nagham Nafiz Hendi*


## Abstract

Cardiovascular diseases (CVD) represent a substantial global health burden, leading to significant morbidity and mortality rates. However, the efficacy and safety of CVD therapies are markedly influenced by individual variability in drug responses and adverse reactions, often attributable to genetic factors. This chapter discusses how pharmacogenomics impacts the safety and efficacy of cardiovascular therapies through advanced genetic testing methods, like genome-wide association studies, polygenic risk scores, and multi-omics analyses. Additionally, the chapter addresses challenges and future perspectives, with a focus on the role of artificial intelligence and machine learning in integrating pharmacogenomics and genotype-based personalized interventions into the routine CVD care to improve long-term health outcomes.


**Keywords:** pharmacogenomics, cardiovascular therapies, gene polymorphisms, precision medicines, genome-wide association studies

## 1. Introduction

Cardiovascular diseases (CVD) remain the leading cause of global disability and mortality, responsible for about 38% of all deaths and straining healthcare systems. These disorders influence the heart and blood circulations, including coronary heart disease, peripheral arterial disease, cerebrovascular disease, and other conditions [1]. However, the response to CVD drugs varies significantly among individuals, leading to suboptimal outcomes and potential adverse reactions. Genetics plays a vital role in drug response variability, with specific CVD therapies showing up to 90% dependence on genetic factors [2]. Given the multifactorial nature of CVD, which involves genetic, environmental, and lifestyle influences, precise and personalized therapeutic strategies become essential for effective management [3].

In recent years, pharmacogenomics has emerged as a promising approach in cardiovascular therapy, offering new opportunities for safe and effective targeted therapies. The field of pharmacogenomics focuses on understanding how genetic variations influence an individual's response to medications. Genetic variations primarily alter cardiovascular drug's concentration (pharmacokinetics), mechanism of action (pharmacodynamics), and the underlying mechanism of CVD [2]. By identifying the genetic factors affecting drug metabolism, receptor interactions, and signaling pathways, pharmacogenomics paves the way for tailored cardiovascular treatment regimens aligned with an individual's genetic profile [4]. This holds particular significance due to the widespread prevalence of CVD, affecting approximately 523 million individuals [1].

The significant advancements in genome-wide association studies (GWAS) and 'omic' technologies, such as proteomics, metabolomics, and transcriptomics, have identified numerous genetic loci linked to cardiovascular conditions, deepening our understanding of the genetic basis of CVD [5, 6]. This information has facilitated pharmacogenomics research, bringing us closer to the goal of precision medicine in managing the global health challenges caused by these diseases [7]. This chapter focuses on utilizing genetic information to optimize standard cardiovascular therapy and improve patient outcomes. It provides comprehensive discussions on key cardiovascular pharmacogenomics, including antithrombotic (antiplatelets and anticoagulants), lipid-lowering agents (statins), and antihypertensive treatments (beta-blockers, angiotensin-converting enzyme inhibitors (ACEI), angiotensin II receptor blockers (ARBs), vasodilators, and diuretics), along with future directions in this field.

## 2. Cardiovascular pharmacogenetics

The influence of genetic makeup on individual response to cardiovascular medications has gained substantial recognition. By 2023, genetic information had been integrated into the Food and Drug Administration (FDA, https://www.fda.gov/drugs/science-and-research-drugs/table-pharmacogenomic-biomarkers-drug-labeling) approved labeling for around 15 cardiovascular treatments. The Clinical Pharmacogenetics Implementation Consortium (CPIC, https://cpicpgx.org/genes-drugs/) [8] and Dutch Pharmacogenetics Working Group (DPWG, https://www.knmp.nl/dossiers/farmacogenetica) [9] provide authoritative guidance through the Pharmacogenomics Knowledgebase (PharmGKB, https://www.pharmgkb.org) on integrating genetics into drug prescribing [10]. These organizations offer evidence-based guidelines for specific gene-drug pairs, optimizing pharmacotherapy decisions in the clinical practice. CPIC and PharmGKB categorize evidence from A (strong) to D (limited/conflicting) [8, 10]. CPIC has issued level A guidelines for several cardiovascular drugs, including clopidogrel, warfarin, and simvastatin [8]. **Table 1** provides an overview of pharmacogenetic biomarkers and clinical recommendations derived from prevalent guidelines for cardiovascular medications.

### 2.1 Antiplatelets

Anti-platelet therapy stands as a cornerstone in managing CVDs, effectively preventing thrombotic incidents of acute coronary syndromes (ACS) and post-percutaneous coronary intervention (PCI) [11]. Gene polymorphisms potently influence various individual responses to this treatment, encompassing acetylsalicylic acid (aspirin), thienopyridine derivatives (clopidogrel, ticlopidine, ticagrelor, and prasugrel), and GP IIb/IIIa receptor inhibitors (tirofiban, lamifiban, epifibatide, and abciximab) [12].

Acetylsalicylic acid modifies cyclooxygenase (COX1) activities to lower thromboxane A2 levels and prevent platelet aggregation. Despite acetylsalicylic acid use,

*DOI: http://dx.doi.org/10.5772/intechopen.113236*

| Medications | Biomarker | SNP ID | Genotype | Effect on response/ safety | Clinical recommendations | Guideline |
|---|---|---|---|---|---|---|
| **Antiplatelets** | | | | | | |
| Acetylsalicylic acid (Aspirin) & abciximab | *PTGS1* | rs3842787 | T | Reduce response | Monitor for thrombosis in patients with resistance. | PharmGKB |
| | *PTGS2* | rs20417 | C | | | |
| | *GPIIIa PlA* | rs2317676 | AG | Reduce response & increase CVE | Consider higher doses of Aspirin & abciximab. | |
| | *ITGA2* | rs1126643 | CT/TT | Reduce response | Limited evidence & require further validation. | — |
| | | rs1062535 | AA/AG | | | |
| | *CYP2C9* | — | *1 | Increase response | Consider lower doses of Aspirin & abciximab. | CPIC |
| | | rs4244285 | *2 | | | |
| | | rs4986893 | *3 | | | |
| | *P2Y1R* | rs1065776 | TT/CT | | Limited evidence & require further validation. | PharmGKB |
| Clopidogrel | *CYP2C19* | rs4244285 | *2 | Reduce response & increase CVE | Consider alternative antiplatelet agents, such as prasugrel or ticagrelor. | CPIC, DPWG, & FDA "Black Box" |
| | | rs4986893 | *3 | | | |
| | | rs3758581 | *17 | Increase response & AE (bleeding risk) | Limited evidence & require further validation. | |
| | | rs28399504 | *4 | Reduce response & increase CVE | | |
| | | rs56337013 | *5 | | | |
| | | rs72552267 | *6 | | | |
| | | rs72558186 | *7 | | | |
| | | rs41291556 | *8 | | | |
| | | rs17884712 | *9 | | | |
| | | rs140278421 | *10 | | | |
| | | rs6413438 | *22 | | | |

| Medications | Biomarker | SNP ID | Genotype | Effect on response/ safety | Clinical recommendations | Guideline |
|---|---|---|---|---|---|---|
| | | rs118203757 | *24 | | | |
| | | rs12769205 | *35 | | | |
| | *ABCB1* | rs1045642 | AA/AG | | Inconsistent & require further validation especially on adverse CVE. | PharmGKB |
| | *PON1* | rs662 | TT | | | CPIC |
| | *CYP3A5* | rs776746 | *3 | Inconsistent effect | Require further validation. | CPIC |
| | *CYP2C9* | rs1799853 | *2 | Reduce response | Limited evidence & require further validation. | CPIC |
| | | rs1057910 | *3 | Reduce response & increase CVE | | CPIC |
| Prasugrel & ticagrelor | *CYP2C19* | rs3758581 | *17 | Increase response & AE (bleeding risk) | | DPWG & FDA |
| | *CYP3A4* | rs35599367 | *22 | Inconsistent effect | | — |
| | *CYP4F2* | rs3093135 | TT | Inconsistent reduce response & increase CVE (MI & CAS) | | |
| | *SLCO1B1* | rs113681054 | C | Inconsistent increase response | | |
| **Anticoagulants** | | | | | | |
| Warfarin | *CYP2C9* | rs1799853 | *2 | Increase response & AE | Consider lower warfarine dose & more frequently INR monitoring. | CPIC, DPWG, & FDA |
| | | rs1057910 | *3 | | | |
| | | rs12777823 | *8 | | Consider 15–30% lower warfarine dose & more frequently INR monitoring in African. | |
| | | rs56165452 | *4 | | | |
| | | rs28371686 | *5 | | | |
| | | rs9332131 | *6 | | | |
| | | rs28371685 | *11 | | | |
| | *CYP2C19* | rs11188082 | T | | | — |

| Medications | Biomarker | SNP ID | Genotype | Effect on response/ safety | Clinical recommendations | Guideline |
|---|---|---|---|---|---|---|
| | *CYP4F2* | rs2108622 | *3 | Reduce response | Consider 5–10% higher warfarine dose in European & Asian. | CPIC |
| | *VKORC1* | rs9923231 | TT | Increase response & AE (bleeding risk) | Consider lower warfarine dose & more frequently INR monitoring. | CPIC, DPWG, & FDA |
| | | rs749671 | G | | | |
| | | rs7294 | CT/TT | | | |
| | | rs9934438 | AG/GG | | | |
| Acenocoumarol | *CYP2C9* | rs1799853 | *2 | Increase response & AE | Consider lower acenocoumarol dose & more frequently INR monitoring, especially with NSAID. | |
| | *CYP4F2* | rs2108622 | *3 | Reduce response | Consider higher acenocoumarol dose. | DPWG |
| | *VKORC1* | rs9923231 | AG/GG | Increase response & AE (bleeding risk) | Consider 50% lower acenocoumarol dose & more frequent INR monitoring, especially with NSAID. | |
| Heparin | *ITGB3, FCGR2A, TDAG8, PTPRJ, IL10, KIR2DS5, HLA-DRA, HLA-DR*3* | — | — | Increase risk of heparin-induced thrombocytopenia | Limited evidence & require further validation. | PharmGKB |
| Direct oral anticoagulants (apixaban, dabigatran, edoxaban, & rivaroxaban) | *ABCB1* | rs4148738 | CT/TT | Reduce response & increase CVE (thromboembolism) | | |
| | | rs1045642 | AA | | | |
| | *CES1* | rs2244613 | GT/TT | Increase response AE (bleeding risk) | | |
| | *AGT* | rs699 | TT | Reduce response | | |
| | *PRKCQ* | rs500766 | CT/TT | Reduced AE | | |
| | *ETV6* | rs2724635 | AA/AG | | | |

| Medications | Biomarker | SNP ID | Genotype | Effect on response/ safety | Clinical recommendations | Guideline |
|---|---|---|---|---|---|---|
| | *CYP3A4, CES1, SLCO1B1, ABCG2, & SULT* | — | — | Increase response & AE | Avoid combining this medication with potent CYP3A4/5 inhibitors, require further validation. | FDA |
| **Lipid-lowering agents** | | | | | | |
| Pravastatin | *KIF6* | rs20455 | AA/GA | Increase response & reduce CVE | Limited evidence & require further validation. | PharmGKB |
| | *SLCO1B1* | rs4149015 | *17 | Increase response & AE (statin-induced myopathy) | Consider patient genotyping prior to dosing with lowering the initial dose. | CPIC, DPWG, & FDA |
| | | rs2306283 | | | | |
| | | rs4149056 | | | | |
| Atorvastatin, simvastatin, rosuvastatin, pravastatin, & lovastatin, pitavastatin | | rs4149056 | *5 | | | |
| | | rs2306283 | *14 | | | |
| | | rs4363657 | | | | |
| | | rs4149056 | | | | |
| | | rs2306283 | *3 | | | |
| | | rs11045819 | | | | |
| Fluvastatin | | rs4149056 | | | | |
| | *CYP2C9* | rs1057910 | *3 | Increase response | CPIC guidelines now cover fluvastatin dosing. | CPIC |
| Atorvastatin, simvastatin, rosuvastatin, pravastatin, & lovastatin, pitavastatin | *CYP3A5* | rs776746 | *3 | Inconsistent effect | Limited evidence & require further validation. | PharmGKB |
| | *CYP3A4* | rs35599367 | *22 | | | |
| | | rs55951658 | *4 | | | |
| | | rs4986910 | *3 | Reduce response | | |
| | | rs2740574 | *1B | | | |
| | | rs2242480 | *1G | | | |
| | *CYP3A7* | rs45446698 | G | | | |

| Medications | Biomarker | SNP ID | Genotype | Effect on response/ safety | Clinical recommendations | Guideline |
|---|---|---|---|---|---|---|
| | *ABCB1* | rs1128503 | AA | Increase response | | |
| | | rs2032582 | | | | |
| | | rs1045642 | | | | |
| | *ABCG2* | rs2231142 | CC | | Consider lower statin dose, alternatives, or combination therapy (e.g., statin + ezetimibe). | CPIC |
| | *UGT1A* | rs887829 | *2 | Reduce response | Limited evidence & require further validation. | PharmGKB |
| | *HMGCR* | rs17244841 | AT | Reduce response | | |
| | *CLMN* | rs8014194 | A | Variable (increase) response | | |
| | *APOE* | rs429358 | E4 | Increase response & reduce CVE | | |
| | | rs7412 | E2 | | | |
| | *CETP* | rs708272 | AA | Reduce response & increase CVE | | |
| **Beta-blockers** | | | | | | |
| Atenolol, bisoprolol, carvedilol, metoprolol, nebivolol, & propranolol | *ADRB1* | rs1801252 | AG/GG | Reduce response & increase CVE | Limited evidence & require further validation. | PharmGKB |
| | | rs1801253 | | | | |
| | *ADRB2* | rs1042713 | GG | | | |
| | | rs1042714 | CG/GG | | | |
| | | rs1800888 | AA | | | |
| | *ADD1* | rs4961 | GT/TT | Increase response & reduce CVE | | |
| | *NPPA* | rs5065 | GG | | | — |
| | | rs4149601 | AA | | | PharmGKB |
| | | rs292449 | CG/GG | | | |

| Medications | Biomarker | SNP ID | Genotype | Effect on response/ safety | Clinical recommendations | Guideline |
|---|---|---|---|---|---|---|
| | *NEDD4L* | rs75982813 | AG/GG | | | |
| | *GRK5* | rs2230345 | TT/AT | Increase response & reduce CVE | | |
| | *CYP2D6* | rs1135840 | GG | Increase response & AE (bradycardia) | | FDA |
| | *CYP2D6* | rs1065852 | AG/GG | Reduce response | | |
| **Direct-acting vasodilators** | | | | | | |
| Hydralazine, minoxidil, & sodium nitroprusside | *NAT2* | — | *4 | Reduce response | Limited evidence & require further validation. | PharmGKB |
| | | rs1801280 | *5D | Increase response & AE (lupus-like symptoms) | | |
| | | rs1799930 | *6B | | | |
| | | rs1799931 | *7A | | | |
| | | rs1801279 | *14B | | | |
| **Renin-angiotensin system inhibitors** | | | | | | |
| ACEI (saptopril, enalapril, & lisinopril) | *ACE* | rs4646994 | DD | Reduce response & increase CVE (mortality) | Limited evidence & require further validation. | PharmGKB |
| | *AGT* | rs699 | AA | Reduce response & increase CVE (blood pressure) | | |
| | *PRKCQ* | rs500766 | CC | Increase AE (angioedema) | | |
| | *ETV6* | rs2724635 | GG | | | |
| ARBs (candesartan, losartan, & olmesartan) | *AGTR1* | rs5186 | AA | Increase response | | |
| **Diuretics** | | | | | | |
| Aldosterone antagonist (Spironolactone) | *ADD1* | rs4961 | GG/GT | Increase response & reduce CVE (MI) | Limited evidence & require further validation. | PharmGKB |
| Loop diuretics (Furosemide) | | | | | | |

| Medications | Biomarker | SNP ID | Genotype | Effect on response/ safety | Clinical recommendations | Guideline |
|---|---|---|---|---|---|---|
| Thiazide diuretics (Hydrochlorothiazide, Chlorthalidone & indapamide) | *NPPA* | rs5065 | GG | | | |
| | | rs4149601 | CC/CG | Increase response | | |
| | | rs292449 | | | | |
| | *NEDD4L* | rs75982813 | AG/GG | | | |
| | *PRKCA* | rs16960228 | A | | | |
| | *YEATS4* | rs7297610 | CC | | | |
| **Antiarrhythmics** | | | | | | |
| Amiodarone, flecainide, sotalol | *KCNE1* | rs1805128 | T | Increase AD (DITdP risk) | Limited evidence & require further validation. | PharmGKB |
| | *SCN5A* | rs7626962 | GT/TT | Reduce response & increase CVE (arrhythmias) | | |
| | *NOS1AP* | rs10919035 | T | Increase AD (ventricular arrhythmia & QT prolongation risk) | | |
| Procainamide | *NAT2* | — | — | Increase response & AE | | FDA |
| Amiodarone, Sotalol flecainide, quinidine, & propafenone | *PITX2* | rs10033464 | GT/TT | Reduced response & CVE (atrial fibrillation recurrence) | | PharmGKB |
| | *ADRB1* | rs1801253 | CC | Increase response | | |
| Quinidine & propafenone | *CYP2D6 & CYP3A4* | — | — | Increase risk (pro-arrhythmia) | Consider patient genotyping prior to dosing with lowering the initial dose. | DPWG & FDA |

*The sources of drug-gene interactions are from common pharmacogenomic guidelines, including PharmGKB (https://www.pharmgkb.org), CPIC (Clinical Pharmacogenetics Implementation Consortium, https://cpicpgx.org/genes-drugs/), DPWG (Dutch Pharmacogenetics Working Group, https://www.knmp.nl/dossiers/farmacogenetica), & FDA (U.S. Food & Drug Administration, https://www.fda.gov/drugs/science-&-research-drugs/table-pharmacogenomic-biomarkers-drug-labeling). Abbreviations: CVE, cardiovascular events; AE, adverse effect; DITdP, drug-induced Torsade de Pointes; MI, myocardial infarction; SNP, single nucleotide polymorphism.*

**Table 1.**
*Pharmacogenomics and clinical recommendations of cardiovascular medications based on common guidelines.*

resistance leads to thrombosis in 5–57% of patients [13]. Notably, two specific variants in the genes encoding COX1 and COX2, rs3842787 in prostaglandin-Endoperoxide Synthase (*PTGS1*) and rs20417 in *PTGS2* affect thromboxane B2 levels [14–16]. The *ITGB3* gene encoding glycoprotein (GP)IIIa harbors different variants (Pro33Leu, rs2317676GG/AG) that necessitate higher aspirin and abciximab doses and augment major ischemic incidents [14]. Genetic variants in *ITGA2* encoding the glycoprotein Ia (GPIa) (rs1126643 and rs1062535) heighten platelet reactivity [16], while the purinergic (*P2RY1*) receptor variant (rs1065776TT/CT, C893T) reduces platelet aggregation [14]. These genetic insights underscore aspirin's complexity in patients' outcomes.

The prodrug clopidogrel, a widely used medication, is metabolized and activated by hepatic cytochrome P450 (CYP) enzymes, majorly CYP2C19, CYP3A5, and CYP3A4 (**Figure 1**) [12]. A widely observed loss-of-function variant of *CYP2C19**2, rs4244285, has been linked to diminished treatment responses and attenuated anti-platelet effects through genome-wide association studies. Individuals with homozygous loss-of-function alleles, such as CY2C19*2/*2, display a complete lack of enzyme functionality and poor metabolism compared to those with reference CY2C19*1/*1 or heterozygous CY2C19*1/*2 alleles, which show extensive or intermediate metabolism [17]. This polymorphism is most prevalent among Asian, African, and European populations, constituting approximately 33%, 18%, and 17% of their respective allele frequencies (**Table 2**) [18].

Other rare loss-of-function alleles, namely *CYP2C19* (*3, rs4986893), (*4, rs28399504), (*5, rs56337013), (*6, rs72552267), (*7, rs72558186), (*8, rs41291556), (*9, rs17884712), (*10, rs6413438), (*22, rs140278421), (*24, rs118203757), and (*35, rs12769205), along with *CYP2C9* (*3, rs1057910) and (*2, rs1799853) have also been identified with uncertain impact, necessitating further validation [19]. Conversely, a gain-of-function variant in the *CYP2C9* (*17, rs3758581) has significantly correlated with elevated enzyme functionality, rapid metabolism, and bleeding risk [20]. This

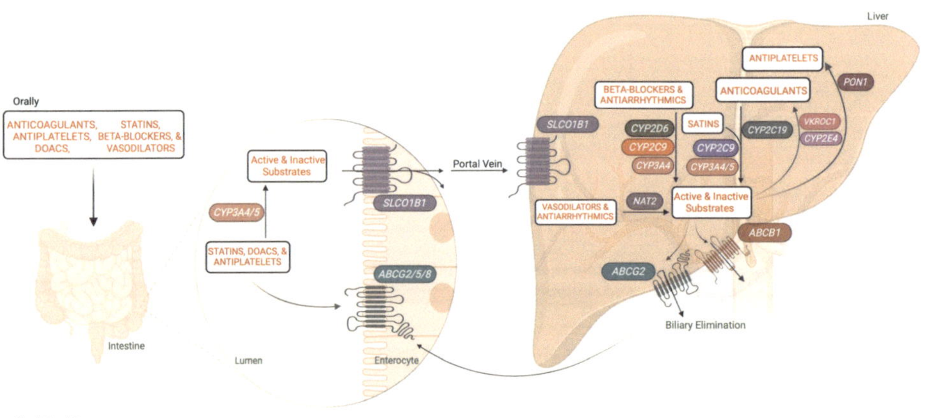


**Figure 1.**
*Pharmacogenetic associations supported by clinical evidence with cardiovascular medications. The pharmacokinetic and pharmacodynamic of cardiovascular medications, including antiplatelets, anticoagulants, DOACs, statins, beta-blockers, direct-acting vasodilators (vasodilators), and antiarrhythmics, are influenced by genetic variations within essential genes. These genes include members of cytochrome P450 family (*CYP2C9, CYP2C19, CYP3A5, CYP4F2, *and* CYP2D6*), as well as* PON1, VKORC1, SLCO1B1, ABCG2, *and* NAT2. *The illustration is generated with BioRender.com.*

| Gene | SNP ID | Consequences | Allele frequency in different populations | | | | | | HGVSc | Functional role |
|---|---|---|---|---|---|---|---|---|---|---|
| | | | Global | African | European | American | South Asian | Middle Eastern | | |
| *ABCB1* | rs4148738 | Intron | 0.611 | 0.770 | 0.540 | 0.603 | 0.403 | 0.570 | ENST00000622132.5: c.2482-2236G>T | Transports molecules and drugs across cellular membranes. |
| | rs1045642 | Missense | 0.572 | 0.797 | 0.469 | 0.568 | 0.411 | 0.519 | ENST00000622132.5: c.3435T>G | |
| *ABCG2* | rs2231142 | Missense | 0.000 | 0.000 | 0.000 | 0.000 | 0.000 | 0.000 | ENST00000237612.8: c.421C>G | |
| *ADD1* | rs4961 | Missense | 0.169 | 0.079 | 0.194 | 0.182 | 0.189 | 0.127 | ENST00000683351.1: c.1378G>A | Part of the cytoskeleton and regulates ion transport, mainly in renal cells. |
| *ADRB1* | rs1801253 | Missense | 0.696 | 0.592 | 0.732 | 0.776 | 0.738 | 0.624 | ENST00000369295.4: c.1165G>A | Mediates the physiological effects of the epinephrine and norepinephrine, mainly in heart. |
| | rs1801252 | Missense | 0.167 | 0.227 | 0.130 | 0.216 | 0.125 | 0.067 | ENST00000369295.4: c.145A>G | |
| *ADRB2* | rs1800888 | Missense | 0.009 | 0.002 | 0.014 | 0.013 | 0.004 | 0.025 | ENST00000305988.6: c.491C T | Regulates specific and rapid signaling by the G protein-coupled receptor and gene transcription. |
| | rs1042714 | Stop gained | 0.682 | 0.821 | 0.632 | 0.757 | 0.794 | 0.760 | ENST00000305988.6: c.79G>T | |
| | rs1042713 | Missense | 0.426 | 0.494 | 0.372 | 0.435 | 0.442 | 0.402 | ENST00000305988.6: c.46G>A | |
| *AGTR1* | rs5186 | 3 prime UTR | 0.206 | 0.063 | 0.296 | 0.258 | 0.081 | 0.206 | ENST00000349243.8: c.*86A>C | Regulates the cardiovascular effects of angiotensin II. |
| *APOE* | rs7412 | Missense | 0.078 | 0.105 | 0.079 | 0.042 | 0.037 | 0.045 | ENST00000252486.9: c.526C>T | Critical for the catabolism of atherogenic lipoprotein constituents. |
| | rs429358 | Missense | 0.157 | 0.215 | 0.138 | 0.112 | 0.105 | 0.067 | ENST00000252486.9: c.388T>C | |
| *CES1* | rs2244613 | Intron | 0.769 | 0.755 | 0.816 | 0.760 | 0.592 | 0.740 | ENST00000360526.8: c.1171-33C>T | Regulates drugs hydrolysis or transesterification. |
| *CETP* | rs708272 | Intron | 0.385 | 0.264 | 0.435 | 0.419 | 0.461 | 0.402 | ENST00000200676.8: c.118 + 279G>A | Transfer cholesteryl ester from high density lipoprotein (HDL) to other lipoproteins. |
| *CTBP2P2* | rs12777823 | Downstream gene | 0.190 | 0.250 | 0.151 | 0.141 | 0.334 | 0.095 | — | A transcriptional repressor, regulates epithelial to mesenchymal transition. |

| Gene | SNP ID | Consequences | Allele frequency in different populations | | | | | | HGVSc | Functional role |
|---|---|---|---|---|---|---|---|---|---|---|
| | | | Global | African | European | American | South Asian | Middle Eastern | | |
| *CYP2C19* | rs72558186 | Splice donor | — | — | — | — | — | — | ENST00000371321.9: c.819 + 2T>A | Catalyze drug metabolism and synthesis reactions. |
| | rs72552267 | Missense | 0.000 | 0.000 | 0.000 | 0.001 | 0.000 | 0.000 | ENST00000371321.9: c.395G>A | |
| | rs6413438 | Missense | 0.001 | 0.003 | 0.000 | 0.001 | 0.000 | 0.000 | ENST00000371321.9: c.680C>T | |
| | rs56337013 | Missense | 0.000 | 0.000 | 0.000 | 0.000 | 0.000 | 0.000 | ENST00000371321.9: c.1297C>T | |
| | rs4986893 | Stop gained | 0.003 | 0.000 | 0.000 | 0.001 | 0.005 | 0.000 | ENST00000371321.9: c.636G>A | |
| | rs4244285 | Synonymous | 0.168 | 0.177 | 0.148 | 0.130 | 0.331 | 0.087 | ENST00000371321.9: c.681G>A | |
| | rs41291556 | Missense | 0.002 | 0.000 | 0.003 | 0.001 | 0.001 | 0.000 | ENST00000371321.9: c.358T>C | |
| | rs3758581 | Missense | 0.952 | 0.987 | 0.937 | 0.953 | 0.886 | 0.927 | ENST00000371321.9: c.991A>C | |
| | rs28399504 | Start lost | 0.002 | 0.001 | 0.003 | 0.006 | 0.001 | 0.000 | ENST00000371321.9: c.1A>G | |
| | rs17884712 | Missense | 0.004 | 0.012 | 0.000 | 0.001 | 0.000 | 0.000 | ENST00000371321.9: c.431G>A | |
| | rs140278421 | Missense | 0.000 | 0.000 | 0.000 | 0.000 | 0.000 | 0.000 | ENST00000371321.9: c.557G>A | |
| | rs12769205 | Intron | 0.173 | 0.197 | 0.148 | 0.133 | 0.330 | 0.092 | ENST00000371321.9: c.332-23A>G | |
| | rs118203757 | Missense | 0.000 | 0.001 | 0.000 | 0.000 | 0.000 | 0.000 | ENST00000371321.9: c.1004G>A | |
| | rs11188082 | Intron | 0.910 | 0.840 | 0.930 | 0.940 | 0.890 | 0.916 | ENST00000371321.9: c.820-12218A>C | |
| *CYP2C9* | rs1799853 | Missense | 0.088 | 0.024 | 0.127 | 0.098 | 0.039 | 0.136 | ENST00000260682.8: c.430C>T | |

DOI: http://dx.doi.org/10.5772/intechopen.113236

| Gene | SNP ID | Consequences | Allele frequency in different populations | | | | | | HGVSc | Functional role |
|---|---|---|---|---|---|---|---|---|---|---|
| | | | Global | African | European | American | South Asian | Middle Eastern | | |
| | rs1057910 | Missense | 0.049 | 0.013 | 0.066 | 0.049 | 0.114 | 0.073 | ENST00000260682.8: c.1075A>C | |
| *CYP2D6* | rs1135840 | Missense | 0.577 | 0.643 | 0.559 | 0.490 | 0.552 | 0.621 | ENST00000645361.2: c.1457G>C | |
| | rs1065852 | Missense | 0.191 | 0.125 | 0.223 | 0.153 | 0.168 | 0.114 | ENST00000645361.2: c.100C>T | |
| *CYP3A4* | rs4986910 | Missense | 0.005 | 0.001 | 0.007 | 0.002 | 0.000 | 0.000 | ENST00000651514.1: c.1334T>C | |
| | rs35599367 | Intron | 0.032 | 0.009 | 0.049 | 0.025 | 0.009 | 0.016 | ENST00000651514.1: c.522-191C>T | |
| | rs2242480 | Intron | 0.310 | 0.732 | 0.094 | 0.358 | 0.346 | 0.228 | ENST00000651514.1: c.1026 + 12G>A | |
| *CYP3A5* | rs776746 | Intron | 0.729 | 0.305 | 0.931 | 0.780 | 0.699 | 0.880 | ENST00000222982.8: c.219-237A>G | |
| *CYP3A7* | rs45446698 | Upstream gene | 0.026 | 0.010 | 0.036 | 0.028 | 0.014 | 0.022 | — | |
| *CYP4F2* | rs3093135 | Intron | 0.151 | 0.136 | 0.166 | 0.154 | 0.156 | 0.174 | ENST00000221700.11: c.344-979T>A | |
| | rs2108622 | Missense | 0.229 | 0.099 | 0.286 | 0.258 | 0.402 | 0.395 | ENST00000221700.11: c.1297G>C | |
| *ETV6* | rs2724635 | Intron | 0.556 | 0.396 | 0.621 | 0.661 | 0.493 | 0.669 | ENST00000396373.9: c.34-5411G>A | Maintenance hematopoiesis and vascular network development. |
| *GRK5* | rs2230345 | Missense | 0.086 | 0.261 | 0.013 | 0.045 | 0.068 | 0.047 | ENST00000392870.3: c.122A>T | Phosphorylates the active G protein-coupled receptors, with unclear mechanisms in cardiovascular diseases. |
| *ITGB3* | rs2317676 | 3 prime UTR | 0.096 | 0.133 | 0.073 | 0.087 | 0.118 | 0.165 | ENST00000559488.7: c.*713A>G | Regulates platelet function |
| *KCNE1* | rs1805128 | Missense | — | — | — | — | — | — | ENST00000399286.3: c.253G>A | Modulates potassium ions flow through ear and cardiac channels. |
| *KIF6* | rs20455 | Missense | 0.489 | 0.798 | 0.361 | 0.386 | 0.445 | 0.443 | ENST00000287152.12: c.2155T>C | Transport cellular intracellular transport of protein complexes. |

| Gene | SNP ID | Consequences | Allele frequency in different populations | | | | | | HGVSc | Functional role |
|---|---|---|---|---|---|---|---|---|---|---|
| | | | Global | African | European | American | South Asian | Middle Eastern | | |
| *PITX2* | rs10033464 | Downstream gene | 0.859 | 0.819 | 0.904 | 0.817 | 0.782 | 0.908 | — | Guiding the development of asymmetric cardiac morphology. |
| *NAT2* | rs1801280 | Missense | 0.382 | 0.305 | 0.447 | 0.352 | 0.338 | 0.452 | ENST00000286479.4: c.341T>C | Catalyzes the acetylation, and thus, activation of drugs. |
| | rs1801279 | Missense | 0.024 | 0.083 | 0.000 | 0.011 | 0.000 | 0.003 | ENST00000286479.4: c.191G>A | |
| | rs1799931 | Missense | 0.041 | 0.033 | 0.026 | 0.096 | 0.074 | 0.048 | ENST00000286479.4: c.857G>A | |
| | rs1799930 | Missense | 0.273 | 0.259 | 0.292 | 0.207 | 0.366 | 0.287 | ENST00000286479.4: c.590G>A | |
| *NEDD4L* | rs75982813 | Upstream gene | 0.063 | 0.091 | 0.061 | 0.041 | 0.037 | 0.032 | — | Regulates the surface expression of renal epithelial sodium channels by ubiquitin-mediated endocytosis and lysosomal targeting. |
| | rs4149601 | Intron | 0.321 | 0.344 | 0.335 | 0.263 | 0.189 | 0.326 | ENST00000400345.8: c.49-16229G>A | |
| | rs292449 | Intron | 0.421 | 0.514 | 0.343 | 0.462 | 0.444 | 0.440 | ENST00000400345.8: c.123-17578G>C | |
| *NOS1AP* | rs10919035 | Intron | 0.198 | 0.214 | 0.147 | 0.214 | 0.265 | 0.204 | ENST00000361897.10: c.178-13122C>G | Modulates intracellular calcium, and up-regulated in dystrophic cardiomyopathy. |
| *P2RY1* | rs1065776 | Synonymous | 0.309 | 0.675 | 0.149 | 0.240 | 0.216 | 0.209 | — | Regulate platelet aggregation. |
| *PON1* | rs662 | Missense | 0.420 | 0.670 | 0.280 | 0.423 | 0.390 | 0.338 | ENST00000222381.8: c.575A>T | Degrades oxidized lipids in LDL, potentially delaying atherosclerosis. |
| *PRKCA* | rs16960228 | Intron | 0.128 | 0.309 | 0.046 | 0.109 | 0.039 | 0.060 | ENST00000413366.8: c.1854 + 3730G>A | Regulator heart contractility |
| *PRKCQ* | rs500766 | Intron | 0.298 | 0.377 | 0.273 | 0.248 | 0.276 | 0.348 | ENST00000263125.10: c.319-1132G>A | Phosphorylate proteins that regulate heart functions and rates. |
| *PTGS1* | rs3842787 | Missense | 0.082 | 0.132 | 0.066 | 0.033 | 0.017 | 0.041 | ENST00000362012.7: c.50C>T | Modulates angiogenesis in endothelial cells. |

| Gene | SNP ID | Consequences | Allele frequency in different populations | | | | | | HGVSc | Functional role |
|---|---|---|---|---|---|---|---|---|---|---|
| | | | Global | African | European | American | South Asian | Middle Eastern | | |
| *PTGS2* | rs20417 | Upstream gene | 0.201 | 0.334 | 0.158 | 0.180 | 0.164 | 0.220 | — | Regulates prostagland synthesis, and functions as a dioxygenase and peroxidase. |
| *SCN5A* | rs7626962 | Missense | 0.000 | 0.000 | 0.000 | 0.000 | 0.000 | 0.000 | ENST00000423572.7: c.3305C>T | Initiates sodium upstroke of the action potential in the heart. |
| *SLCO1B1* | rs4363657 | Intron | 0.182 | 0.148 | 0.171 | 0.177 | 0.088 | 0.193 | ENST00000256958.3: c.1498-1331T>A | Regulates the sodium-independent uptake of different molecules and drugs. |
| | rs4149056 | Missense | 0.121 | 0.032 | 0.159 | 0.130 | 0.049 | 0.206 | ENST00000256958.3: c.521T>C | |
| | rs2306283 | Missense | 0.532 | 0.768 | 0.402 | 0.560 | 0.516 | 0.477 | ENST00000256958.3: c.388A>C | |
| | rs113681054 | Intergenic | 0.183 | 0.153 | 0.171 | 0.181 | 0.093 | 0.199 | — | |
| *UGT1A4* | rs887829 | Intron | 0.361 | 0.449 | 0.321 | 0.324 | 0.410 | 0.339 | ENST00000373409.8: c.868-7110C>T | Catalyze drug metabolism and synthesis reactions. |
| *VKORC1* | rs9934438 | Intron | 0.319 | 0.100 | 0.378 | 0.391 | 0.179 | 0.513 | ENST00000394975.3: c.174-136C>T | Reduces of inactive vitamin K 2,3-epoxide to active vitamin K in the endoplasmic reticulum membrane. |
| | rs9923231 | Upstream gene | 0.319 | 0.100 | 0.370 | 0.390 | 0.178 | 0.519 | — | |
| | rs749671 | Upstream gene | 0.316 | 0.099 | 0.374 | 0.388 | 0.178 | 0.472 | — | |
| | rs7294 | 3 prime UTR | 0.403 | 0.458 | 0.383 | 0.400 | 0.712 | 0.250 | ENST00000394975.3: c.*134G>A | |
| *YEATS4* | rs7297610 | Intergenic | 0.124 | 0.303 | 0.063 | 0.072 | 0.022 | 0.079 | — | Involves in transcriptional activation. |

*The allele frequencies of genes associated with the pharmacogenomic of cardiovascular medications are identified using the Genome Aggregation Database (gnomAD, https://gnomad.broadinstitute.org, accessed on September 5th, 2023), and annotated using the Ensembl Effect Predictor release 108 (VEP, https://grch37.ensembl.org/index.html, accessed on September 4th, 2023). Abbreviations: HGVSc, Human Genome Variation Society sequence nomenclature descriptions from Ensembl; SNP, single nucleotide polymorphism, AF; allele frequency.*

**Table 2.**
*Functions of cardiovascular genetic factors and their allele frequencies among diverse populations.*

variant exhibit minor allele frequencies of 0.3, 0.93, and 0.98 in Caucasian, European, and African populations, respectively (**Table 2**) [18]. However, the uncertain clinical implications for carriers of *17 necessitate additional research due to inconsistent findings.

Genetic polymorphisms in the *CYP2C19* gene markedly impact enzymatic activity and link to adverse cardiovascular events, including mortality, myocardial infarction (MI), and stroke [17]. Consequently, the Food and Drug Administration (FDA) issued a "Black Box" warning for clopidogrel, suggesting *CYP2C19* genotyping and the consideration of alternative antiplatelet agents before prescribing antiplatelet therapies for PCI or ACS patients with a high risk of poor responses, as also recommended by CPIC and DPWG [9].

CYP3A4, CYP2C19, and CYP2B6 primarily activate Prasugrel, while CYP3A4 activates ticagrelor's active metabolite [12]. Clinical trials indicate better cardiovascular event risk reduction with ticagrelor and prasugrel than clopidogrel in ACS [21]. Polymorphisms in the ATP-binding cassette B1 (*ABCB1*, rs1045642) and paraoxonase 1 (*PON1*, rs662) genes lower clopidogrel bioavailability, with inconsistent impact on adverse cardiovascular outcomes. Clinical guidelines exclude *ABCB1* or *CYP2C19* variants for prasugrel or ticagrelor [22]. However, those agents have higher bleeding rates, costs, and discontinuation [12]. Genetic variants, including *CYP3A4* (*22, rs35599367), *CYP3A5* (*3, rs776746), *CYP4F2* (rs3093135), *CYP2C19* (*17, rs3758581), and solute carrier organic anion transporter 1B1 (*SLCO1B1*, *rs113681054*) [23, 24], may impact prasugrel and ticagrelor antiplatelet outcomes, necessitating further research.

## 2.2 Anticoagulants

Oral anticoagulants, particularly Vitamin K antagonists and direct-acting oral anticoagulants (DOACs), are critical in preventing and treating thromboembolic disorders [12]. These medications have achieved significant success in cardiovascular therapeutics through candidate genes and GWAS investigations [25, 26].

### *2.2.1 Vitamin K antagonists*

The narrow therapeutic index for Vitamin K antagonists, such as warfarin and acenocoumarol, necessitates close monitoring of the international normalized ratio (INR). This monitoring ensures the achievement of optimal anticoagulation within the INR range of 2–3 and prevents hemorrhage [27]. The metabolism (inactivation) of warfarin occurs predominantly in the liver through CYP2C9, with minimal involvement of CYP4F2. These therapeutic agents function as inhibitors of the vitamin K epoxide reductase complex-1 (VKORC1), subsequently impeding the biological activation of vitamin K1. VKORC1 activates coagulation factors by enhancing Vitamin K reduction, thus disrupting the biological activation of vitamin K1 (**Table 2**) [12].

Common genotypes, particularly *CYP2C9* (*3, rs1057910), (*2, rs1799853), and rs9332238, have been detected as key contributors to variability in dose requirements of warfarin, accounting for around 50% [28]. Individuals carrying loss-of-function alleles of *CYP2C9* are at elevated risk of hemorrhagic consequences and demand reduced warfarin dosages [26]. GWAS have additionally linked the *3 allele (rs2108622, V433M) variant in *CYP4F2* as a distinct factor influencing variability in warfarin dosing. *CYP4F2* plays a role in metabolizing vitamin K1, acting alongside *VKORC1* to prevent excessive vitamin K accumulation [29]. In European and Asian populations, the *3 allele requires 5–10% higher warfarin doses than the *1 allele.

However, this association is absent within African populations where *CYP2C9**8 (rs12777823) and the *CYP2C19* intron variant (rs11188082) are predominant, primarily due to disparities in allele frequencies [25].

Genetic mutations in the promoter region of *VKORC1*, commonly rs9923231 (1639G>A), rs9934438 (1173T>C), rs749671, and rs7294 (3730G>A), impact the hepatic abundance of *VKORC1* mRNA transcripts and the sensitivity of warfarin [26]. Individuals with reduced *VKORC1* expression levels require less warfarin doses, whereas those with gain-of-function mutations require higher doses to maintain a steady anticoagulant effect. Numerous uncommon variations in *VKORC1* with non-synonymous alterations (defined as alterations to the protein's amino acid sequence) have been associated with warfarin resistance and heightened dosage requirements [30].

Pharmacogenomics of warfarin underscores the significant role of genetic heritage on drug responses. Asian individuals often demand reduced amounts due to the prevalence of *VKORC1* loss-of-function variants, while increased doses are needed for African individuals because gain-of-function *VKORC1* variants are more prevalent. Among individuals of African ancestry, there are additional *CYP2C9* variants (*5, rs28371686; *6, rs28371686; *8, rs9332131; and *11, rs28371685 alleles) that reduce warfarin dose requirements by 15–30% and are more common than *2 and *3 alleles compared to Caucasians (**Table 2**) [31]. The Clarification of Optimal Anticoagulation through Genetics (COAG) trial underscored that ignoring these genetic variations resulted in warfarin overdosing in African Americans [32].

Acknowledging the significance of these genetic patterns, the FDA has updated drug packaging to include dosage instructions that consider pharmacogenetic testing of *CYP2C9* and *VKORC1* genotypes. The CPIC and DPWG guidelines recommend this therapeutic approach before initiating warfarin treatment in pediatrics and adults. Studies showed that genotype-guided early warfarin treatment shortened stabilization time, improved cost-effect anticoagulation, and led to better clinical outcomes [33].

Acenocoumarol, a coumarin derivative, is primarily utilized to prevent instances of thromboembolism and deep vein thrombosis, with its effectiveness influenced by genetic polymorphisms in the *CYP2C9*2* rs1799853, *CYP4F2*3* rs2108622, and *VKORC1* (rs9923231, 1639G>A) genes. Several algorithms predict dosage requirements of acenocoumarol based on genetic factors, ethnicity, and demographic data, such as Verde et al.'s "acenocoumarol-dose genotype score" [34–36]. DPWG guidelines emphasize close INR monitoring during non-steroidal anti-inflammatory drug (NSAID) changes for those with specific genetic profiles on acenocoumarol. The *VKORC1* genotype significantly impacts dosing variability, although precise recommendations remain limited due to rigorous monitoring requirements [37].

### *2.2.2 Heparin*

Heparin-induced thrombocytopenia (HIT) is a dangerous immune reaction to heparin anticoagulants. Predicting HIT is challenging due to limited confirmed cases and genetic complexity. Studies have inconsistently identified risk genes associated with HIT-related clotting, such as integrin beta 3 (*ITGB3,* encodes GPIIIa), Fc gamma receptor IIa (*FCGR2A*), T-cell death-associated gene-8 (*TDAG8*), protein tyrosine phosphatase receptor type J (*PTPRJ*, also known as CD148), interleukin 10 (*IL10*), and human leukocyte antigen DR (*HLA-DRA*) [38–42].

A GWAS identified a substantial association of missense genetic variant near the *TDAG8* with elevated platelet factor 4/heparin antibodies, even in non-heparin-treated patients [43]. Candidate genomic study determined a strong link between the *HLA-DRB3**01:01 allele and a higher risk of HIT. They also noted an interaction between the killer cell immunoglobulin like receptor 2 domains, short cytoplasmic tail 5 (*KIR2DS5*) and the *HLA-C1 KIR* binding group. This suggests that HLA variations and CD4+ T cells might play a role in HIT development, pending confirmation through functional assays [38]. Furthermore, comprehensive multiethnic studies with confirmed HIT cases are needed to identify genomic biomarkers for effective preventive strategies.

### *2.2.3 Direct oral anticoagulants*

DOACs, like apixaban, dabigatran, edoxaban, and rivaroxaban, have gained popularity due to their advantageous pharmacokinetics and pharmacodynamics, eliminating the need for regular INR monitoring. However, instances of varied plasma DOAC levels and increased hemorrhagic risks have enhanced pharmacogenomic research [27]. Plasma level variation mainly arises from drug interactions and genetics, particularly depending on the absorption and activation functions of intestinal P-glycoprotein, coded by the adenosine triphosphate (ATP)-binding cassette B1 transporter/multidrug resistance-1 (*ABCB1/MDR1*) gene, and hepatic carboxylesterase 1 (*CES1*) [12].

The *ABCB1* polymorphisms (such as rs1045642 and rs4148738) and *CES1* polymorphism (rs2244613) inconsistently affect dabigatran levels [44]. Plasma levels of rivaroxaban and apixaban were associated significantly with genetic variations in *CYP3A4*, *ABCB1*, ATP Binding Cassette G2 (*ABCG2*), and sulfotransferase (*SULT*), while edoxaban linked to *CYP3A4*, *CES1*, *SLCO1B1*, and *ABCB1* [45]. The FDA recently advises against combining this medication with potent CYP3A4/5 inhibitors, like carbamazepine, phenobarbital, phenytoin, or rifampin, as well as inducers, such as boceprevir, itraconazole, and clarithromycin [46]. Exploring these genetic factors, particularly in elderly patients with multiple conditions and concurrent medications, is crucial for understanding drug-gene interactions.

## 2.3 Lipid-lowering agents

The high occurrence of CVD, obesity, and metabolic syndrome necessitates the utilization of statins, a class of drugs known as 3-hydroxy-3-methylglutaryl-coenzyme A reductase (HMGCR) inhibitors, including atorvastatin, rosuvastatin, simvastatin, pravastatin, fluvastatin, lovastatin and pitavastatin [47]. Statins effectively decrease total and low-density lipoprotein (LDL) cholesterol levels by up to 55%, leading to a 20–30% reduction in cardiovascular events. The clinical response to statin treatment varies significantly among individuals. Approximately one-third of individuals achieve insufficient desired LDL reductions, with rare yet severe adverse consequences to the medication, including myopathy and rhabdomyolysis. Genetic variations linked to cholesterol synthesis, absorption, and transport can impact the effectiveness of statin therapy alongside environmental influences and patient adherence. Genomic studies identified genes associated with lipid metabolisms, such as apolipoprotein E (*APOE*), apolipoprotein B (*APOB*), cholesteryl ester transfer protein (*CETP*), LDL receptor (*LDLR*), cholesterol transport, such as *ABCG5/8*, *ABCG2*, *ABCB1/MDR1*, kinesin-like protein 6 (*KIF6*), solute carrier organic anion transporter 1B1 (*SLCO1B1*), calmin (*CLMN*), and CYP450 metabolizing enzymes family [47].

The utilization of simvastatin, a prominent HMGCR inhibitor, has faced a decline attributed to its link to myopathy risk in about 28% of patients [48]. This risk exhibits a dose-dependent pattern, prompting regulatory measures by the FDA to restrict the maximum allowable dose [49]. GWAS suggest a link between *SLCO1B1* genetic variations, including rs4149056 (c388A-c521C), rs2306283 (388A>G), and noncoding rs4363657 (c.1498-1331T>C), and statin-induced myopathy, including simvastatin and atorvastatin. These polymorphisms reduce the function of the organic anion transporting polypeptides B1 (*OATP1B1*) found on hepatocytes' sinusoidal membrane, leading to increased circulating levels of simvastatin active form. GWAS revealed a threefold elevated risk associated with each C genotype, particularly in homozygous individuals. Carriers of *SLCO1B1**5 allele have a 4- to 5-fold higher risk of severe creatine kinase-positive statin-induced myopathy and a 2- to 3-fold higher risk of creatine kinase-negative myopathy [50].

Variations in the *CYP3A4* gene have been connected to different responses to statin treatment, including simvastatin, atorvastatin, and lovastatin. Individuals carrying the homozygous/heterozygous *CYP3A4*22* (rs35599367) or homozygous *CYP3A5*3* (rs776746) polymorphisms, along with *CYP3A4*4* (rs55951658) haplotype on statin therapy exhibit an escalated response that decreased total and LDL cholesterol levels [51, 52]. Conversely, those with the missense *CYP3A4*3* (rs4986910, M445T), *CYP3A4* promoter polymorphism (rs2740574, A290G), or *CYP3A4*1*G haplotype (rs2242480) might not achieve the anticipated lipid-lowering effects from statins [53–55]. One GWAS on the plasma level of atorvastatin identified associations with polymorphisms near *CYP3A7* (rs45446698) and UDP Glucuronosyltransferase-1A (*UGT1A*, rs887829) [56]. Studies suggest that genetic variability in *CYP2C9**3 (rs1057910) is connected to elevated levels of fluvastatin [57].

The *ABCB1* genetic polymorphisms influence the efficacy of simvastatin, with less common variants (rs1128503, 1236T; rs2032582, 2677 non-G; and rs1045642, 3435T) occurring in patients who experience muscle-related side effects [58]. The pharmacokinetics of atorvastatin and rosuvastatin are affected through variants in the *ABCG2* gene, which encodes breast cancer resistance protein (BCRP) transporter. Individuals with the CC genotype at rs2231142 experience more significant reductions in LDL cholesterol levels compared to those with AA genotypes [59].

In some studies, kinesin-like protein 6 (KIF6), involved in intracellular transport, has been linked to coronary artery disease. These studies suggest potential statin benefits for carriers of the rs20455 (Trp719Arg) missense polymorphism in the *KIF6* gene [60]. However, a meta-analysis of 19 studies discovered an inconsistent link between this polymorphism and nonfatal coronary artery disease [61]. The *CLMN* polymorphism, rs8014194, explains only 1% of statin response variability, with carriers experiencing notably greater reductions in total cholesterol. Initial GWAS suggest that the *APOE* E2 (rs7412) (526C>T) and E4 (rs429358, 388T>C) alleles might significantly reduce the LDL levels and lower instances of nonfatal myocardial infarction and mortality when treated with lipid-lowering therapy [62]. However, support for these associations varies across all studies [63].

Pharmacogenetic research has focused on the *CETP* gene, particularly examining the *TaqIB* variant, rs708272. Individuals with a B1B1 genotype on statin treatment experience slower coronary artery disease progression than B2B2 carriers. While some studies, including Boekholdt et al.'s meta-analysis, find no connection between the TaqIB polymorphism and pravastatin treatment [64], the Regression Growth Evaluation Statin Study (REGRESS) revealed potential pharmacogenetic interactions. This study identified higher 10-year mortality in male statin-treated patients with the *B2* allele, compared to those with the B1B1 genotype (**Table 1**) [65]. In the future, there is an expectation of a more comprehensive understanding of statins' function and the individual variations in response.

Consequently, clinical guidelines suggest adjusting simvastatin and atorvastatin dosages according to the *SLCO1B1* genotype, although the significance has diminished due to the availability of safer statins, such as rosuvastatin and or pravastatin [66]. The FDA has eliminated the requirement for further confirmatory testing of *SLCO1B1*-simvastatin genotyping [67]. CPIC guidelines now cover rosuvastatin dosing based on *ABCG2* and *SLCO1B1* genotypes and fluvastatin dosing based on *CYP2C9* genotype [66]. This expansion to high-intensity statins, including atorvastatin and rosuvastatin, is expected to enhance the use of pharmacogenetic-guided approaches for selecting and dosing statins in clinical practice.

### 2.4 Beta-blockers

Beta-blockers function through competitive antagonism of endogenous catecholamines at the beta-1 and beta-2 adrenergic receptors, encoded by *ADBR1* and *ADBR2*, in the heart and blood vessels. These medications are commonly prescribed to reduce heart rate, lower blood pressure, and enhance survival and left ventricular ejection fraction following an MI, including atenolol, bisoprolol, carvedilol, metoprolol, nebivolol, propranolol. However, the response to beta-blockers can vary significantly among individuals due to genetic factors influencing the pharmacokinetics (*CYP2D6*) and the pharmacodynamics (*ADBR1*, *ADBR2*, and *GRK5*).

Genetic variants of *ADBR1*, commonly rs1801252 (Ser49Gly) and rs1801253 (Arg389Gly), have been linked to impaired down-regulation and altered signal transduction *in vitro* [68, 69]. Associations of Gly49 are linked to more significant reductions in the end diastolic diameter than the Ser49 genotype. Moreover, Ser49 carriers have higher heart rates and increased mortality than Gly49 carriers on beta-blocker treatment [70]. Clinical research indicates that individuals with homozygous Arg389 genotype tend to respond more positively to beta-blockers, enhancements in the left ventricular ejection fraction (LVEF), and overall risk reduction of hospitalizations and mortality compared to Gly389 [71, 72]. However, this correlation and reports of improved beta-blocker response on blood pressure and heart rate demonstrated inconsistency [73, 74].

Prevalent polymorphisms in the *ADBR2*, mainly rs1042713 (Arg16Gly), rs1042714 (Gln27Gly), and rs1800888 (Thr164Ile), have shown increased adenylyl cyclase activity, leading to enhanced agonist-induced downregulation of *ADBR2* [75]. However, associations of these variants with cardiovascular outcomes are inconsistent. Most studies observed no link between these genetic variants and cardiovascular improvement [76], but smaller studies suggested the Glu27 allele might be associated with higher LVEF than the Gln27 allele when using beta-blockers [77]. A prevalent four amino-acid deletion (Del322-325) reduces alpha(2C)-AR (*ADRA2C*) activity in cells and associates with adverse heart failure outcomes [78], though it did not affect the beta-blocker Evaluation of Survival Trial (BEST) with bucindolol [72].

The CYP2D6 enzyme predominantly metabolizes carvedilol, metoprolol, nebivolol, propranolol, and timolol. CYP2D6 is unnecessary for metabolizing other beta-blockers, like atenolol, bisoprolol, and nadolol. Common genetic variants of *CYP2D6* lead to a range of phenotypes, varying from increased enzyme function due to gene duplication to complete loss of function. Such as homozygous rs1135840 and rs1065852, caused by gene deletion or splicing defects [79]. Approximately, 5–10% of the population carries two or more *CYP2D6* alleles, such as the *4 allele, with reduced activity. This raises the circulating levels of beta-blockers, leading to substantial blood pressure and heart rate reduction and a greater risk of adverse drug reactions [80]. Although *CYP2D6* variations seem to affect heart rate response to beta-blockers, their significant influence on blood pressure response and cardiovascular risk reduction remains uncertain [81].

The G protein-coupled receptor kinase 5, encoded by *GRK5*, is an intracellular component that attenuates signaling from beta-adrenergic receptors. The rs2230345 (Gln41Leu) variant heightens *GRK5* activity, mimicking the impact of a beta-blocker [82]. Those with the 41Leu variant show improved heart failure and hypertension outcomes, potentially reducing beta-blockers effectiveness [83]. This could favor alternative medications depending on the medical condition. Nevertheless, further research is needed to establish the clinical implications of these variants for guiding beta-blocker therapy.

Considering the established pharmacogenomic interactions of beta-blockers and *ADBR1* polymorphisms, utilizing multiple risk alleles could enhance the strategic management of this therapy [84]. Genetic variations in *CYP2D6* might impact beta-blocker pharmacokinetics, but application in prescribing is limited. The FDA-approved metoprolol label downplays the impact of CYP2D6-dependent metabolism on safety but advises caution with potent CYP2D6 inhibitors, such as quinidine, fluoxetine, paroxetine, and propafenone [85]. The DPWG guidance suggests tailored dosing, including gradual titration for intermediate and poor metabolizers and considering alternatives, like bisoprolol, for ultra-rapid metabolizers as needed [9].

### 2.5 Direct-acting vasodilators

Direct-acting vasodilators decrease blood pressure by relaxing vascular smooth muscle, including hydralazine, minoxidil, and sodium nitroprusside. Hydralazine is recommended for secondary hypertension treatment and primarily undergoes hepatic metabolism by N-acetyltransferase type 2 (NAT2). Genetic variants *in NAT2* determine acetylation rates, with *NAT2*4* indicating rapid acetylation, and the common *5 rs1801280 (341T>C), *6 rs1799930 (590G>A), *7 rs1799931 (857G>A), and the rare *14 rs1801279 (191G>A) suggesting slower rates [86]. Rapid acetylators have lower hydralazine exposure, affecting blood pressure response. Slow acetylators might experience more potent antihypertensive effects due to increased drug exposure [87], potentially elevating the risk of rare adverse reactions, like lupus-like symptoms [88]. Nonetheless, the evidence supporting *NAT2* genotyping for predicting hydralazine's safety and efficacy remains inconclusive.

### 2.6 Renin-angiotensin system inhibitors

Renin-angiotensin system (RAS), including ACEIs (such as captopril, enalapril, and lisinopril) and ARBs (such as candesartan, losartan, and olmesartan) serves as a cornerstone in the management of CVD, encompassing hypertension, ACS, heart failure, and nephropathy. Polymorphisms in renin-angiotensin-aldosterone-related genes, particularly *ACE*, angiotensinogen (*AGT*), and angiotensin-II receptors I and II (*AGTR1* and *AGTR2*), can potentially impact the ACEIs and ARBs mechanisms. Individuals with DD homozygosity of the *ACE* insertion/deletion rs4646994

(287-Alu) variant exhibit elevated *ACE* activity in both plasma and tissues, which is associated with higher 10-year mortality rates [89]. Around 10% of patients on ACEIs developed a dry cough, likely caused by an accumulation of bradykinin during therapy. Studies have linked this cough to the ACE insertion/deletion variant and a specific polymorphism in the bradykinin B2 (*B2R*) gene's promoter region [90].

The *AGT* rs699 (Met235Thr) allele carriers tend to have elevated angiotensin levels, which may be connected to increased blood pressure [91]. The *AGTR1* rs5186 (A1166C) polymorphism has been studied for its beneficial influence on ARB response [92]. A GWAS identified two moderately associated variants in the protein kinase C theta (*PRKCQ*, rs500766) and ETS transcription 6 (*ETV6*, rs2724635), genes involved in immune regulation related to ACEI-induced angioedema [93]. Current evidence lacks definitive pharmacogenomic associations between *ACE*, *AGT*, or *AGT1R* polymorphisms and the effectiveness and safety of ACEIs or ARBs. The inconsistent results and study limitations undermine the reliability of these findings, warranting further research to improve precision medicine guidance.

## 2.7 Diuretics

Thiazide diuretics (such as hydrochlorothiazide, chlorthalidone, and indapamide) play a crucial role in managing hypertension, while loop diuretics (such as bumetanide, ethacrynic acid, and furosemide) and aldosterone antagonist (like spironolactone) are the preferred choice for addressing fluid retention in heart failure.

Research suggests that individuals carrying the rs4961 (Gly460>Trp) variant in the α-adducin gene (*ADD1*) exhibit more favorable blood pressure responses to thiazide, loop, and spironolactone diuretics, revealing an association with salt sensitivity [94]. Carriers of the Trp460 variant experience a more pronounced protective effect, approximately 38%, against heart attacks (MI) and strokes compared to individuals with the Gly460 genotype [95]. The *NPPA* rs5065 (T2238C) variants, encode atrial natriuretic peptide, showed that C allele carriers had lower CVD risk and more significant blood pressure reductions with chlorthalidone than amlodipine. However, those with the TT genotype had a higher risk of heart attack, stroke, and all-cause mortality with chlorthalidone [96].

Furthermore, genetic variations in the *NEDD4L* (rs4149601, rs292449, and rs75982813, encodes neural precursor cell expressed developmentally downregulated 4-like enzyme), *PRKCA* (rs16960228, encodes Protein kinase C alpha), and *YEATS4* (rs7297610, encodes YEATS Domain Containing-4) consistently show a significant link to cardiovascular outcomes with thiazide diuretics (**Table 1**) [97–99]. Despite their potential, these gene variations have not yet impacted diuretic prescriptions due to conflicting research. Further studies may lead to personalized diuretic therapies for hypertension and related conditions.

## 2.8 Antiarrhythmics

Antiarrhythmic drugs block the potassium current channel (IKr) and prolong QT intervals, increasing the drug-induced Torsade de Pointes (DITdP) malignant arrhythmia risk, including amiodarone, flecainide, procainamide, and sotalol. Some common gene variants have been linked to DITdP, constituting around 10% of cases known as congenital long QT syndrome (cLQTS) incomplete penetrance. The rs1805128 (D85N) polymorphism in potassium voltage-gated channel E1 (*KCNE1*), encoding Ikr subunit, and rs7626962 (S1103Y) sodium voltage-gated Channel Alpha 5 (*SCN5A*), encoding cardiac sodium channel, exhibit a strong connection to DITdP development [100, 101]. A significant SNP, rs10919035, in nitric oxide synthase 1 adaptor protein (*NOS1AP*), is notably prevalent in amiodarone related TdP cases and associated with ventricular arrhythmia and QT prolongation [102].

Prevalent polymorphisms at the 4q25 locus near the *PITX2* gene, rs10033464, have been linked to an increased risk of atrial fibrillation (AF) and reduced responsiveness to certain antiarrhythmic drugs (**Table 1**) [103]. Additionally, a genetic variant rs1801253 in *ADRB1* (Arg389Gly) is associated with better outcomes with rhythm control strategies for managing AF [104]. CYP2D6 and CYP3A4 metabolize some antiarrhythmic drugs as beta-blockers, such as flecainide, quinidine, and propafenone. Limited evidence suggests that genetic variations in *CYP2D6* and *CYP3A4* may impact their pharmacokinetics and affect the QTc interval, as indicated by their classification in PharmGKB as level 2A and in CPIC level as B-C [105, 106].

Clinical studies use a QT alert system to monitor high-risk DITdP patients. A polygenic risk score of common variants shows potential for enhancing personalized prevention and guiding AF treatment based on an individual's genotype [107]. The FDA label for procainamide highlights response differences based on acetylation speed by *NAT2* but does not mention any specific genotype for acetylation status determination. The FDA recommends caution with quinidine and propafenone in individuals with *CYP2D6* and *CYP3A4* inhibitions due to high adverse effects risk, like pro-arrhythmia. Although there are no specific CPIC guidelines for these drugs, the DPWG recommends reducing the standard doses by 50% and 30% in *CYP2D6* poor metabolizers (**Table 1**) [37].

## 3. Future perspectives in personalized cardiovascular therapy

Advancements in pharmacogenomics offer significant potential for personalized cardiovascular therapy, leveraging an individual's genetic profile. High-throughput genotyping and next-generation sequencing technologies enhance our understanding of how genetics influence responses to cardiovascular drugs [108]. Integrating pharmacogenomic data into electronic health records enhances clinical decision-making, promising safer and more cost-effective medication regimens. Notably, genetic markers identified through GWAS, and multi-omics analyses enable personalized selection of antiplatelets, statins, and warfarin dosages, reducing the occurrence of adverse cardiovascular events [9, 17, 22, 33, 66].

Following the validation of identified polymorphisms, the transformative genetic approach revolutionizes cardiovascular therapy, including implementing polygenic risk scores. However, cardiovascular pharmacogenomics faces challenges due to patient variability and limited study sizes. These challenges encompass genetic data diversity limitations, difficulties in clinical integration, technical and sociopolitical constraints, and the complexity of genetic interactions. Addressing these issues necessitates collaborative efforts, supported by artificial intelligence and machine learning, to uncover polygenic predictors and fully realize the potential of precision medicine in complex CVDs with multiple drug regimens, like heart failure [109]. While logistical challenges persist in obtaining early genotype results, the prospect of pre-emptive or point-of-care testing offers potential solutions.

## 4. Conclusion

Substantial evidence underscores genetic associations with efficacy and tolerance of cardiovascular therapies, including antiplatelets, anticoagulants, lipid-lowering agents, and, to moderate extent, beta-blockers. Pharmacogenetic testing has become a standard practice, enhancing cardiovascular treatment outcomes. However, further research is necessary to guide genotype-based drug selection and validate genetic variation's effect on drug responses and safety among different populations. Ultimately, precision medicine aims to prove its superiority of genotype-based personalized interventions over current standard care and improve overall health outcomes.

## Conflict of interest

The authors declare no conflict of interest.

## Author details

Georges Nemer and Nagham Nafiz Hendi*
Division of Genomics and Translational Biomedicine, College of Health and Life Sciences, Hamad Bin Khalifa University, Doha, Qatar

*Address all correspondence to: nhendi@hbku.edu.qa

## References

[1] Roth GA et al. Global burden of cardiovascular diseases and risk factors, 1990-2019: Update from the GBD 2019 study. Journal of the American College of Cardiology. 2020;**76**(25):2982-3021

[2] Matthaei J et al. Heritability of metoprolol and torsemide pharmacokinetics. Clinical Pharmacology and Therapeutics. 2015;**98**(6):611-621

[3] Watkins WS et al. De novo and recessive forms of congenital heart disease have distinct genetic and phenotypic landscapes. Nature Communications. 2019;**10**(1):4722

[4] Roden DM et al. Opportunities and challenges in cardiovascular pharmacogenomics: From discovery to implementation. Circulation Research. 2018;**122**(9):1176-1190

[5] Khera AV et al. Genome-wide polygenic scores for common diseases identify individuals with risk equivalent to monogenic mutations. Nature Genetics. 2018;**50**(9):1219-1224

[6] Reel PS et al. Machine learning for classification of hypertension subtypes using multi-omics: A multi-Centre, retrospective, data-driven study. eBioMedicine. 2022;**84**:104276

[7] Mensah GA et al. Emerging concepts in precision medicine and cardiovascular diseases in racial and ethnic minority populations. Circulation Research. 2019; **125**(1):7-13

[8] Relling MV et al. The clinical pharmacogenetics implementation consortium: 10 years later. Clinical Pharmacology and Therapeutics. 2020; **107**(1):171-175

[9] Lee CR et al. Clinical pharmacogenetics implementation consortium guideline for CYP2C19 genotype and clopidogrel therapy: 2022 update. Clinical Pharmacology and Therapeutics. 2022;**112**(5):959-967

[10] Gong L, Whirl-Carrillo M, Klein TE. PharmGKB, an integrated resource of pharmacogenomic knowledge. Current Protocols. 2021;**1**(8):e226

[11] Powers WJ, Rabinstein AA, Ackerson T, Adeoye OM, Bambakidis NC, Becker K, et al. Correction to: Guidelines for the early management of patients with acute ischemic stroke: 2019 update to the 2018 guidelines for the early management of acute ischemic stroke: A guideline for healthcare professionals from the American Heart Association/ American Stroke Association. Stroke. 2019;**50**(12):e440-e441

[12] Magavern EF, Kaski JC, Turner RM, Drexel H, Janmohamed A, Scourfield A, et al. Corrigendum to: The role of pharmacogenomics in contemporary cardiovascular therapy: A position statement from the European Society of Cardiology Working Group on Cardiovascular Pharmacotherapy. European Heart Journal - Cardiovascular Pharmacotherapy. 2022;**9**(1):116

[13] Liu Q et al. Model based on single-nucleotide polymorphism to discriminate aspirin resistance patients. Stroke and Vascular Neurology. 2023;**16**: svn-2022-002228

[14] Li Q et al. Frequency of genetic polymorphisms of COX1, GPIIIa and P2Y1 in a Chinese population and association with attenuated response to aspirin. Pharmacogenomics. 2007;**8**(6):577-586

[15] Yi X et al. Platelet response to aspirin in Chinese stroke patients is independent of genetic polymorphisms of COX-1 C50T and COX-2 G765C. Journal of

Atherosclerosis and Thrombosis. 2013; **20**(1):65-72

[16] Wang H et al. Association of GPIa and COX-2 gene polymorphism with aspirin resistance. Journal of Clinical Laboratory Analysis. 2018;**32**(4):e22331

[17] Verma SS et al. Genomewide association study of platelet reactivity and cardiovascular response in patients treated with clopidogrel: A study by the international clopidogrel pharmacogenomics consortium. Clinical Pharmacology and Therapeutics. 2020; **108**(5):1067-1077

[18] Ionova Y et al. CYP2C19 allele frequencies in over 2.2 million direct-to-consumer genetics research participants and the potential implication for prescriptions in a large health system. Clinical and Translational Science. 2020; **13**(6):1298-1306

[19] Mega JL et al. Cytochrome p-450 polymorphisms and response to clopidogrel. The New England Journal of Medicine. 2009;**360**(4):354-362

[20] Yadav AK et al. Substantiation of a clopidogrel metabolism-associated gene (CYP2C19) variation among healthy individuals. Indian Heart Journal. 2023; **75**(5):343-346

[21] Claassens DMF et al. A genotype-guided strategy for oral P2Y(12) inhibitors in primary PCI. The New England Journal of Medicine. 2019; **381**(17):1621-1631

[22] Her AY et al. Platelet function and genotype after DES implantation in east Asian patients: Rationale and characteristics of the PTRG-DES consortium. Yonsei Medical Journal. 2022;**63**(5):413-421

[23] Liedes H et al. CYP3A4*22 may increase bleeding risk in ticagrelor users. Basic & Clinical Pharmacology & Toxicology. 2023;**133**(2):202-207

[24] Varenhorst C et al. Effect of genetic variations on ticagrelor plasma levels and clinical outcomes. European Heart Journal. 2015;**36**(29):1901-1912

[25] Asiimwe IG et al. A genome-wide association study of plasma concentrations of warfarin enantiomers and metabolites in sub-Saharan black-African patients. Frontiers in Pharmacology. 2022;**13**:967082

[26] Parra EJ et al. Genome-wide association study of warfarin maintenance dose in a Brazilian sample. Pharmacogenomics. 2015;**16**(11): 1253-1263

[27] Pokorney SD et al. Patients' time in therapeutic range on warfarin among US patients with atrial fibrillation: Results from ORBIT-AF registry. American Heart Journal. 2015;**170**(1):141-148, 148 e1

[28] Wadelius M et al. Association of warfarin dose with genes involved in its action and metabolism. Human Genetics. 2007;**121**(1):23-34

[29] Singh O et al. Influence of CYP4F2 rs2108622 (V433M) on warfarin dose requirement in Asian patients. Drug Metabolism and Pharmacokinetics. 2011; **26**(2):130-136

[30] Scott SA et al. Warfarin pharmacogenetics: CYP2C9 and VKORC1 genotypes predict different sensitivity and resistance frequencies in the Ashkenazi and Sephardi Jewish populations. American Journal of Human Genetics. 2008;**82**(2):495-500

[31] Allabi AC, Gala JL, Horsmans Y. CYP2C9, CYP2C19, ABCB1 (MDR1) genetic polymorphisms and phenytoin metabolism in a Black Beninese

population. Pharmacogenetics and Genomics. 2005;**15**(11):779-786

[32] Kimmel SE et al. A pharmacogenetic versus a clinical algorithm for warfarin dosing. The New England Journal of Medicine. 2013;**369**(24):2283-2293

[33] Johnson JA et al. Clinical pharmacogenetics implementation consortium (CPIC) guideline for pharmacogenetics-guided warfarin dosing: 2017 update. Clinical Pharmacology and Therapeutics. 2017;**102**(3):397-404

[34] Ragia G et al. A novel acenocoumarol pharmacogenomic dosing algorithm for the Greek population of EU-PACT trial. Pharmacogenomics. 2017;**18**(1):23-34

[35] Ragia G, Manolopoulos VG. Pharmacogenomics of anticoagulation therapy: The last 10 years. Pharmacogenomics. 2019;**20**(16): 1113-1117

[36] Verde Z et al. A novel, single algorithm approach to predict acenocoumarol dose based on CYP2C9 and VKORC1 allele variants. PLoS One. 2010;**5**(6):e11210

[37] Yoon DY et al. Pharmacogenomic information from CPIC and DPWG guidelines and its application on drug labels. Translational and Clinical Pharmacology. 2020;**28**(4):189-198

[38] Karnes JH et al. Influence of human leukocyte antigen (HLA) alleles and killer cell immunoglobulin-like receptors (KIR) types on heparin-induced thrombocytopenia (HIT). Pharmacotherapy. 2017;**37**(9):1164-1171

[39] Rollin J et al. Increased risk of thrombosis in FcgammaRIIA 131RR patients with HIT due to defective control of platelet activation by plasma IgG2. Blood. 2015;**125**(15):2397-2404

[40] Harris K, Nguyen P, Van Cott EM. Platelet PlA2 polymorphism and the risk for thrombosis in heparin-induced thrombocytopenia. American Journal of Clinical Pathology. 2008;**129**(2): 282-286

[41] Rollin J et al. Polymorphisms of protein tyrosine phosphatase CD148 influence FcgammaRIIA-dependent platelet activation and the risk of heparin-induced thrombocytopenia. Blood. 2012;**120**(6):1309-1316

[42] Pouplard C et al. Interleukin-10 promoter microsatellite polymorphisms influence the immune response to heparin and the risk of heparin-induced thrombocytopenia. Thrombosis Research. 2012;**129**(4):465-469

[43] Karnes JH et al. A genome-wide association study of heparin-induced thrombocytopenia using an electronic medical record. Thrombosis and Haemostasis. 2015;**113**(4):772-781

[44] Sychev DA et al. The impact of ABCB1 (rs1045642 and rs4148738) and CES1 (rs2244613) gene polymorphisms on dabigatran equilibrium peak concentration in patients after total knee arthroplasty. Pharmacogenomics and Personalized Medicine. 2018;**11**:127-137

[45] Kryukov AV et al. Influence of ABCB1 and CYP3A5 gene polymorphisms on pharmacokinetics of apixaban in patients with atrial fibrillation and acute stroke. Pharmacogenomics and Personalized Medicine. 2018;**11**:43-49

[46] XARELTO (rivaroxaban). 2023. Available from: https://www.accessdata.fda.gov/drugsatfda_docs/label/2011/202439s001lbl.pdf

[47] Hindi NN, Alenbawi J, Nemer G. Pharmacogenomics variability of lipid-

lowering therapies in familial hypercholesterolemia. Journal of Personalized Medicine. 2021;**11**(9):877

[48] Abed W et al. Statin induced myopathy among patients attending the National Center for Diabetes, Endocrinology, & Genetics. Annals of Medicine and Surgery. 2022;**74**:103304

[49] FDA Drug Safety Communication: Revised Dose Limitation for Zocor (Simvastatin) When Taken with Amiodarone. 2011. Available from: https://www.fda.gov/drugs/drug-safety-and-availability/fda-drug-safety-communication-revised-dose-limitation-zocor-simvastatin-when-taken-amiodarone

[50] Mykkanen AJH et al. Genomewide association study of simvastatin pharmacokinetics. Clinical Pharmacology and Therapeutics. 2022; **112**(3):676-686

[51] Elalem EG et al. Association of cytochromes P450 3A4*22 and 3A5*3 genotypes and polymorphism with response to simvastatin in hypercholesterolemia patients. PLoS One. 2022;**17**(7):e0260824

[52] Wang A et al. Ile118Val genetic polymorphism of CYP3A4 and its effects on lipid-lowering efficacy of simvastatin in Chinese hyperlipidemic patients. European Journal of Clinical Pharmacology. 2005;**60**(12):843-848

[53] Thompson JF et al. An association study of 43 SNPs in 16 candidate genes with atorvastatin response. The Pharmacogenomics Journal. 2005;**5**(6): 352-358

[54] Kajinami K et al. CYP3A4 genotypes and plasma lipoprotein levels before and after treatment with atorvastatin in primary hypercholesterolemia. The American Journal of Cardiology. 2004; **93**(1):104-107

[55] Peng C et al. Polymorphisms in CYP450 genes and the therapeutic effect of atorvastatin on ischemic stroke: A retrospective cohort study in Chinese population. Clinical Therapeutics. 2018; **40**(3):469-477 e2

[56] Turner RM et al. A genome-wide association study of circulating levels of atorvastatin and its major metabolites. Clinical Pharmacology and Therapeutics. 2020;**108**(2):287-297

[57] Buzkova H et al. Lipid-lowering effect of fluvastatin in relation to cytochrome P450 2C9 variant alleles frequently distributed in the Czech population. Medical Science Monitor. 2012;**18**(8):CR512-517

[58] Fiegenbaum M et al. The role of common variants of ABCB1, CYP3A4, and CYP3A5 genes in lipid-lowering efficacy and safety of simvastatin treatment. Clinical Pharmacology and Therapeutics. 2005;**78**(5):551-558

[59] Keskitalo JE et al. ABCG2 polymorphism markedly affects the pharmacokinetics of atorvastatin and rosuvastatin. Clinical Pharmacology and Therapeutics. 2009;**86**(2):197-203

[60] Iakoubova OA et al. KIF6 Trp719Arg polymorphism and the effect of statin therapy in elderly patients: Results from the PROSPER study. European Journal of Cardiovascular Prevention and Rehabilitation. 2010;**17**(4):455-461

[61] Assimes TL et al. Lack of association between the Trp719Arg polymorphism in kinesin-like protein-6 and coronary artery disease in 19 case-control studies. Journal of the American College of Cardiology. 2010;**56**(19):1552-1563

[62] Barber MJ et al. Genome-wide association of lipid-lowering response to statins in combined study populations. PLoS One. 2010;**5**(3):e9763

[63] Zintzaras E et al. APOE gene polymorphisms and response to statin therapy. The Pharmacogenomics Journal. 2009;**9**(4):248-257

[64] Boekholdt SM et al. Cholesteryl ester transfer protein TaqIB variant, high-density lipoprotein cholesterol levels, cardiovascular risk, and efficacy of pravastatin treatment: Individual patient meta-analysis of 13,677 subjects. Circulation. 2005;**111**(3):278-287

[65] Regieli JJ et al. CETP genotype predicts increased mortality in statin-treated men with proven cardiovascular disease: An adverse pharmacogenetic interaction. European Heart Journal. 2008;**29**(22):2792-2799

[66] Cooper-DeHoff RM et al. The clinical pharmacogenetics implementation consortium guideline for SLCO1B1, ABCG2, and CYP2C9 genotypes and statin-associated musculoskeletal symptoms. Clinical Pharmacology and Therapeutics. 2022; **111**(5):1007-1021

[67] 23andMe Releases New FDA-Cleared Genetic Report on Simvastatin, a Commonly Prescribed Statin. 2023. Available from: https://investors.23andme.com/news-releases/news-release-details/23andme-releases-new-fda-cleared-genetic-report-simvastatin

[68] Brodde OE. Beta1- and beta2-adrenoceptor polymorphisms and cardiovascular diseases. Fundamental & Clinical Pharmacology. 2008;**22**(2): 107-125

[69] Magnusson Y et al. Ser49Gly of beta1-adrenergic receptor is associated with effective beta-blocker dose in dilated cardiomyopathy. Clinical Pharmacology and Therapeutics. 2005;**78**(3):221-231

[70] Rathz DA et al. Amino acid 49 polymorphisms of the human beta1-adrenergic receptor affect agonist-promoted trafficking. Journal of Cardiovascular Pharmacology. 2002; **39**(2):155-160

[71] Chen L et al. Arg389Gly-beta1-adrenergic receptors determine improvement in left ventricular systolic function in nonischemic cardiomyopathy patients with heart failure after chronic treatment with carvedilol. Pharmacogenetics and Genomics. 2007;**17**(11):941-949

[72] Bristow MR et al. An alpha2C-adrenergic receptor polymorphism alters the norepinephrine-lowering effects and therapeutic response of the beta-blocker bucindolol in chronic heart failure. Circulation. Heart Failure. 2010;**3**(1):21-28

[73] Ma ST et al. Association between beta1 adrenergic receptor gene Arg389Gly polymorphism and risk of heart failure: A meta-analysis. Genetics and Molecular Research. 2015;**14**(2):5922-5929

[74] Li YJ et al. Polymorphisms of Arg389Gly of beta1-adrenergic receptor gene and essential hypertension risk: A meta analysis. Zhonghua Yi Xue Za Zhi. 2011;**91**(44):3115-3119

[75] Al-Balushi K et al. Frequencies of the Arg16Gly, Gln27Glu and Thr164Ile adrenoceptor beta2 polymorphisms among Omanis. Sultan Qaboos University Medical Journal. 2015;**15**(4):e486-e490

[76] de Groote P et al. Association between beta-1 and beta-2 adrenergic receptor gene polymorphisms and the response to beta-blockade in patients with stable congestive heart failure. Pharmacogenetics and Genomics. 2005; **15**(3):137-142

[77] Liu J et al. beta1-adrenergic receptor polymorphisms influence the response to metoprolol monotherapy in patients with essential hypertension. Clinical

Pharmacology and Therapeutics. 2006; **80**(1):23-32

[78] Kardia SL et al. Multiple interactions between the alpha 2C- and beta1-adrenergic receptors influence heart failure survival. BMC Medical Genetics. 2008;**9**:93

[79] Zisaki A, Miskovic L, Hatzimanikatis V. Antihypertensive drugs metabolism: An update to pharmacokinetic profiles and computational approaches. Current Pharmaceutical Design. 2015;**21**(6): 806-822

[80] Bijl MJ et al. Genetic variation in the CYP2D6 gene is associated with a lower heart rate and blood pressure in beta-blocker users. Clinical Pharmacology and Therapeutics. 2009;**85**(1):45-50

[81] Luzum JA et al. CYP2D6 genetic variation and Beta-blocker maintenance dose in patients with heart failure. Pharmaceutical Research. 2017;**34**(8): 1615-1625

[82] Liggett SB et al. A GRK5 polymorphism that inhibits beta-adrenergic receptor signaling is protective in heart failure. Nature Medicine. 2008;**14**(5):510-517

[83] Lobmeyer MT et al. Polymorphisms in genes coding for GRK2 and GRK5 and response differences in antihypertensive-treated patients. Pharmacogenetics and Genomics. 2011;**21**(1):42-49

[84] Petersen M et al. Association of beta-adrenergic receptor polymorphisms and mortality in carvedilol-treated chronic heart-failure patients. British Journal of Clinical Pharmacology. 2011;**71** (4):556-565

[85] LOPRESSOR (metoprolol tartrate). 2020. Available from: https://www.accessdata.fda.gov/drugsatfda_docs/label/2020/018704s027,028lbl.pdf

[86] Spinasse LB et al. Different phenotypes of the NAT2 gene influences hydralazine antihypertensive response in patients with resistant hypertension. Pharmacogenomics. 2014;**15**(2):169-178

[87] Han LW et al. Effect of N-acetyltransferase 2 genotype on the pharmacokinetics of hydralazine during pregnancy. Journal of Clinical Pharmacology. 2019;**59**(12):1678-1689

[88] Schoonen WM et al. Do selected drugs increase the risk of lupus? A matched case-control study. British Journal of Clinical Pharmacology. 2010; **70**(4):588-596

[89] Brugts JJ et al. Genetic determinants of treatment benefit of the angiotensin-converting enzyme-inhibitor perindopril in patients with stable coronary artery disease. European Heart Journal. 2010; **31**(15):1854-1864

[90] Nishio K et al. Angiotensin-converting enzyme and bradykinin gene polymorphisms and cough: A meta-analysis. World Journal of Cardiology. 2011;**3**(10):329-336

[91] Schelleman H et al. Angiotensinogen M235T polymorphism and the risk of myocardial infarction and stroke among hypertensive patients on ACE-inhibitors or beta-blockers. European Journal of Human Genetics. 2007;**15**(4):478-484

[92] Liu Y et al. Association of AGTR1 A1166C and CYP2C9 *3 gene polymorphisms with the antihypertensive effect of valsartan. International Journal of Hypertension. 2022;**2022**:7677252

[93] Pare G et al. Genetic variants associated with angiotensin-converting enzyme inhibitor-associated angioedema. Pharmacogenetics and Genomics. 2013;**23**(9):470-478

[94] Wang R et al. Association between alpha-adducin gene polymorphism (Gly460Trp) and genetic predisposition to salt sensitivity: A meta-analysis. Journal of Applied Genetics. 2010;**51**(1):87-94

[95] Psaty BM et al. Diuretic therapy, the alpha-adducin gene variant, and the risk of myocardial infarction or stroke in persons with treated hypertension. JAMA. 2002;**287**(13):1680-1689

[96] Lynch AI et al. Pharmacogenetic association of the NPPA T2238C genetic variant with cardiovascular disease outcomes in patients with hypertension. JAMA. 2008;**299**(3):296-307

[97] Turner ST et al. Genomic association analysis of common variants influencing antihypertensive response to hydrochlorothiazide. Hypertension. 2013;**62**(2):391-397

[98] McDonough CW et al. Association of variants in NEDD4L with blood pressure response and adverse cardiovascular outcomes in hypertensive patients treated with thiazide diuretics. Journal of Hypertension. 2013;**31**(4):698-704

[99] Duarte JD et al. Association of chromosome 12 locus with antihypertensive response to hydrochlorothiazide may involve differential YEATS4 expression. The Pharmacogenomics Journal. 2013;**13**(3):257-263

[100] Kaab S et al. A large candidate gene survey identifies the KCNE1 D85N polymorphism as a possible modulator of drug-induced torsades de pointes. Circulation. Cardiovascular Genetics. 2012;**5**(1):91-99

[101] Paulussen AD et al. Genetic variations of KCNQ1, KCNH2, SCN5A, KCNE1, and KCNE2 in drug-induced long QT syndrome patients. Journal of Molecular Medicine (Berlin, Germany). 2004;**82**(3):182-188

[102] Jamshidi Y et al. Common variation in the NOS1AP gene is associated with drug-induced QT prolongation and ventricular arrhythmia. Journal of the American College of Cardiology. 2012;**60**(9):841-850

[103] Parvez B et al. Common genetic polymorphism at 4q25 locus predicts atrial fibrillation recurrence after successful cardioversion. Heart Rhythm. 2013;**10**(6):849-855

[104] Parvez B et al. A common beta1-adrenergic receptor polymorphism predicts favorable response to rate-control therapy in atrial fibrillation. Journal of the American College of Cardiology. 2012;**59**(1):49-56

[105] Rouini MR, Afshar M. Effect of CYP2D6 polymorphisms on the pharmacokinetics of propafenone and its two main metabolites. Thérapie. 2017;**72**(3):373-382

[106] Doki K et al. Serum flecainide S/R ratio reflects the CYP2D6 genotype and changes in CYP2D6 activity. Drug Metabolism and Pharmacokinetics. 2015;**30**(4):257-262

[107] Strauss DG et al. Common genetic variant risk score is associated with drug-induced QT prolongation and torsade de pointes risk: A pilot study. Circulation. 2017;**135**(14):1300-1310

[108] Infante T et al. Network medicine: A clinical approach for precision medicine and personalized therapy in coronary heart disease. Journal of Atherosclerosis and Thrombosis. 2020;**27**(4):279-302

[109] Segar MW et al. Phenomapping of patients with heart failure with preserved ejection fraction using machine learning-based unsupervised cluster analysis. European Journal of Heart Failure. 2020;**22**(1):148-158